Wounded & Defined

Trading Victim for Victory

And this is the victory that
conquers the world—our faith.
1 John 5:4 NCV

Courage inspires!
God Bless-
Tonya

Tonya Shellnutt

Wounded & Defined

ISBN: 978-0-578-87789-1

Written by Tonya Shellnutt
Content Development by Robert Noland
Edited by Christy Distler
Design by Amy Balamut

Acknowledgements

I want to give special thanks to ALL the pastors and faith leaders out there who have influenced my life by always sharing TRUTH and the healing power of the Gospel. We live in a day and age where everyone wants to cancel you and the life changing message of Hope you bring. However, when they do, it denies the power of the cross. Please never stop being bold and courageous. You have given me and so many HOPE!

I want to give a special shout-out to one particular pastor who has had such an incredible impact on my life and I am forever grateful for you—Dr. Paul Jones! Thank you for empowering me to overcome my victimhood by clinging to God's truth. You always validated me where I was in my journey, but you never allowed me to wallow in my pity! Love you so much, Brother!!!

I want to thank Robert Noland for taking a chance on this project. Many times I would read the manuscript and wonder how could you even put into words the pain and agony I felt. I know God used your giftedness to bring light out of darkness. I can never thank you enough for your help.

Thank you to my wonderful children for teaching me so much about life, grace, humility, and perseverance. I am thankful for you listening to ALL of my "Life Lesson's by Tonya." I am so proud of you ALL and pray God will continue to show you grace and mercy in your faith journey!

Thank you to my great-grandmother, Laura Irwin, for always sharing your faith and how you overcame so many hardships in life. You shattered glass ceilings and I pray I can be half the woman you were. You taught me to chase my dreams and be courageous.

Lastly, thank you to the most amazing man I have ever known—Rich Shellnutt. Your super-power is LOVE. You have taught me how to love people and always look for the good in people. Thank you for protecting me mostly from my own self-destructive path and for showing me grace and mercy. Thank you for ALWAYS empowering me to chase my dreams. I love you so much!

Contents

The Lord replies,

"I have seen violence done to the helpless,
and I have heard the groans of the poor.
Now I will rise up to rescue them,
as they have longed for me to do."

Psalm 12:5

INTRODUCTION

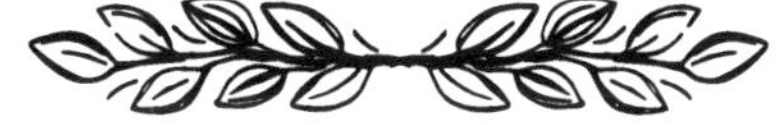

Stolen Innocence

When I was five years old, my parents wanted to go out to party with their friends one evening, a common occurrence in our home. The clock was ticking for their meet-up time, and quickly running out of options for babysitters and desperate to keep their plans for fun, my mom and dad opted for the last resort—an eighteen-year-old boy who lived down the street. They hardly knew him at all. No real connection or relationship to our family. But he was available.

Not long after they had driven away, he took me into my parents' bedroom. He got undressed and demanded I do the same. Confused and terrified, I was completely unable to comprehend why and how a senior in high school would be doing this to a kindergartener. The horrible reality he had planned out was, to be blunt, child rape. My parents' careless, reckless choice for their daughter offered him a crime of opportunity.

Every sense of security I had in my young life was shattered at that moment. With no possible understanding of what he was doing to me, yet still feeling such a violation could only be wrong, I felt a sudden burst of self-preservation kick in. Through the physical pain and emotional shock, I began to kick, punch, and scream, somehow managing to pull away and escape to the bathroom. I frantically slammed the door, locked myself in, and curled up on the cold tile floor as tightly as my little body could manage.

While I recall crying hysterically, lying there in a wide-awake nightmare, that is where my memory of this horrific event goes dark. In that moment in time at just five years old, an enveloping, ominous cloud moved in over my life, creating a devastating sexual imprint that would last for far too many years.

My life had been violated and disrupted by a sick and self-absorbed pedophile. But my personal response was no different from most victims, as shame and guilt took up residence, coupled with questions and fears that cut deep into my young heart, creating gaping wounds. Over time, those festered into painful scars that slowly hardened into a protective armor I relied upon to keep out anyone I deemed could possibly hurt me.

The problem with building your own dysfunctional fortress for all the wrong reasons is, of course, you are constructing an emotional and mental prison for yourself. At the time, I had no idea what was being molded into my impressionable identity, but there began a distorted belief system that cut deep roots into my emotional well-being.

That night, I did not speak a word to my parents about what had happened. While my recollection of the event is savagely clear, some of the details were blocked and blurred. Only victims of such violence can understand that dynamic of clarity and confusion. On some days, the memories are distractingly loud and haunt me, while at other times, they cause me to grieve and mourn for all those who have suffered from sexual abuse.

And many years later, I came to understand firsthand that while sympathy expressed is good, empathy from a heart that has healed of the same tragedy can truly become a catalyst to change someone's life.

CHAPTER ONE

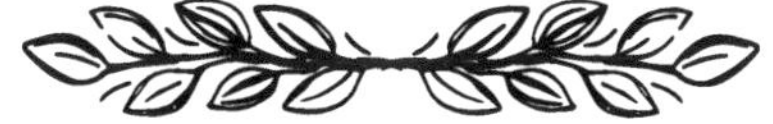

The What-ifs and the Why-Mes

Eventually, we all figure out that there will be some questions in this life that are never going to get answered. My reasons for those uncertainties started early. When I was only six months old, my biological father abandoned my mom and me. Whatever the circumstances that led up to his decision, the bottom line for me as an innocent infant was that I had been deserted by the first man who was supposed to love and care for me.

When I was two years old, my mom married a man named Bill who she had been seeing for a while. He was twice divorced and had two older daughters from one of his previous marriages, but they never lived with us. To his credit, my mother's new husband took me in, providing for me as if I were one of his own. In fact, for years I lived under the assumption that he was my biological father.

Bill worked as a deputy for the local sheriff's department, and a great deal of inherent stress accompanied his career. Most evenings, he would come home carrying the weight of the dark side of humanity he had dealt with on the job, and go straight to the refrigerator to start his nightly marathon of beer drinking. After some particularly difficult days, he would stop at the local bar and have a few there before coming home to continue.

Like so many people, Bill drank to medicate the pain of his own open wounds. His work required an eight-hour focus on other people's problems and bad behavior. That is especially true for anyone who works in law enforcement. Often, maintaining laser focus is the only thing standing between them and death. But then quitting time would shift Bill back to his personal life, and his past failures and current faults would come roaring back to the forefront of his mind and heart.

Mom had her own gaping wounds from her previous life and my birth father's abandonment. But neither she nor Bill ever talked about the past or the pain. Drinking and partying with friends, all in a desperate search for distraction, translated into a booze bash for birthdays, holidays, weddings, funerals, graduations, and sporting events—any excuse to drink with others looking for a good time. But alcohol was always the guest of honor.

Honestly, my mom was not much of a serious drinker, but she wanted to please Bill. So, wherever he went and whatever he wanted to do, she would follow. Being with him meant she was not alone and also meant she knew where he was, what he was doing, and who he was with. All these dynamics in our family led to many of the incidents that would have lasting effects on me. The lack of guidance and protection from my parents created circumstances like the one I described in the introduction.

I have to assume that the shame, guilt, and sheer shock of the crime committed against me silenced my ability to communicate what happened that night. There were so many horrible questions that constantly invaded my mind when my memory would be triggered.

Thoughts like these came randomly: *What if my parents had decided to consider my safety, put me first, and just stay home? What if my mom would have told my dad to go on and she would stay with me? What if my dad had come to his senses and realized they could not possibly leave me alone with a teenage boy they did not know? What if I had managed to escape the house and go to a neighbor to call the police? What if he had been a boy who loved Jesus and showed me what genuine concern and care from a male could be like?*

The vicious cycle of assigning blame was constant. Countless times I asked God to erase those terrible memories and put an end to all the what-ifs. But then those questions eventually ended up back at the forefront of my mind, my thoughts racing with the why-mes.

My nightmare experience as a little girl, coupled with keeping that boy's dirty secret, started me down a bad road of living in a constant mode of self-protection. In my heart, I was terrified of any male, especially if I did not know him. When I walked into my classroom on the first day of third grade and saw my teacher was a man, fear struck me and stayed throughout that year.

During my elementary school days, any time my parents planned their night out and the doorbell rang, if I saw a young man standing there to babysit, to say that I freaked out would be an understatement. Every time, I begged and pleaded with them to not leave me alone with him. In sheer terror and with tears flooding my eyes, I grabbed my mother's leg and held on with a death grip, assuming the horror was about to happen again. My mind screamed, *What if I can't escape behind a locked door this time?*

But my cries were dismissed and overlooked, written off as a little girl "just being dramatic." Amazingly, those traumatic scenes never tipped my parents off to suspect something was actually wrong.

During my childhood years, I suffered from frequent nightmares of a "boogie man" coming after me. The connection is of course easy to make now, but at the time I was not mature enough to understand what was happening in my mind. While some nights were worse than others, few offered peaceful, secure sleep. Not wanting to disturb my parents but not being able to endure being alone, I would often end up in a fetal position on the floor of their room next to the bed, clutching my security blanket.

Our family began to grow again when I was six, as my sister was born. Then just nine months and ten days later, my brother was born. He was seven weeks premature and had to stay in the NICU for quite a while before they brought him home. So now with a half-sister and half-brother, along with Bill's older daughters, my step-sisters, who we saw regularly, I was right in the middle of five children.

A SILENT TSUNAMI

Life brought another blindsiding surprise when I entered the fifth grade. In health class, the teacher began to talk about topics like puberty and the reproduction process. The discussion of our body parts and the introduction of basic sex education opened up a new floodgate to the memories of my abuse. Understanding what had physically happened to me took the trauma to a new depth. The images poured out suddenly, without warning, swallowing me up in a tsunami of pain and misunderstood emotions. I was overcome with a strange mix of guilt and anxiety as the reality of the crime began to sink in for the first time.

Like fighting for air when you're drowning, I vividly recalled my screams and tearful pleading for the violator to stop. Feeling horribly confused, I went home from school and did what I had sworn to myself I would never do: I told my parents what happened on that night five years before.

After I managed to blurt out the sordid details, they appeared concerned yet stayed oddly calm. They asked me a few questions about that night. I answered to the best of my ability, and what happened next made everything far worse. They got up from the table and never spoke another word about the event to me again. No apologies. No reassurances. No support. And so I vowed to never speak of the violation again—at least to them. (In fairness, about five years later, my mom brought up the situation and offered to take me to counseling.)

Now even more confused at the lack of recognition and my parents' silence, I determined the only possible conclusions that might warrant the nature of their response: First, I must have actually been the one in the wrong. Somehow, I must have been responsible for what happened to me. Second, I began to question the reality of the events that night. Had this horror really happened, or had I somehow invented the whole thing?

Locking in on my new target of blame—myself—I once again tried to block the entire nightmare out of my mind. But the flashbacks kept coming with a vengeance. I could not escape. I couldn't make them go away. (And I still struggle to shut them out even today, all these years later.) The shame and fear I felt was so raw and debilitating.

I began to accept my new identity: damaged. I was damaged. How badly? I wasn't sure yet. But when you start to view yourself through such a destructive lens, the degree of the issue doesn't seem to matter anymore. Because now it's not so much about who, what, when, or how; the fact is, you're just . . . damaged.

A few months following my confession, after I had turned eleven, my parents informed me that Bill was not actually my "real dad" but that he was starting the legal process to officially adopt me as his daughter. Wait. So my real dad abandoned me and the father I have always thought was my dad is not actually my dad at all? Just when I start to think life can't get worse, somehow it finds a way to kick me down even farther.

Their confession created an entirely new set of questions to join my others: *Who is my biological father? Why did he leave? What was wrong with me that he would want to give me up at only six months old?* Inside my heart, this revelation created yet another deep layer of guilt and shame. More damage. Then I began to connect the sexual abuse to this new news. What if my birth father had been my dad at five years old? Would the rape have happened? Maybe he would have never allowed that boy into our home? Maybe he would have protected me like fathers should protect their little girls?

This information also brought clarity about my family dynamics. Some questions I'd had for a long time began to make sense now. I had always felt like the odd-man-out with Bill's two older children from his previous marriage and my mom's two kids she had with Bill. I had this strange sense that I didn't belong.

As a smart-mouth, argumentative kid, I was not exactly everyone's little darling anyway. I hated the fact that I knew I was not *anyone's* favorite, because all I ever really wanted was to be loved and accepted—mainly by Bill. The short season after my real dad left and before Bill came along had created the first true bond between me and my mom. I think because of the brief time that she felt it was us against the world, she always did her best to make me feel valued and treasured to some degree.

Bill always had trouble articulating his feelings and expressing affection to anyone. Sometimes he would show a bit of emotion when he had enough to drink. But when sober, he tended to be angry, closed off, and stone-faced.

I felt my best was never good enough for Bill. No matter how well I did or how much I improved at anything, he was always quick to remind me I could do better. While I was very athletic and participated in many sports, Bill rarely attended my games.

He would occasionally show up, but then he would point out anything he deemed I had done wrong, regardless of what my coach said. With my grades, anything above a B was met with silence, while below a B brought only negative attention.

For most young girls and boys faced with this parenting dynamic, the tendency is to either give up or seek perfection, both of which create issues. Being headstrong and the way I was wired in my personality, I chose perfection—a dangerous game when you live with an identity crisis. My pattern was to work harder than ever to win Bill's attention and approval. And the more he stayed away and disapproved when he did come around, the harder I pursued achievement. (Years later, I learned that many sexual abuse victims become extremely performance-based.)

Over time, I came to the false conclusion that who you are is what you do. Maybe a more accurate version would be that I decided that who you are is only as good as what you did *today*. I placed identity and security on an ever-sliding scale of up-to-the-minute performance. That belief became deeply entrenched in my attitude and actions.

All this emotional chaos in my twelve-year-old mind left me wondering what to do with all these feelings of insecurity and insignificance. As the roots of the overwhelming pain grew deeper, the only response I could muster up was to hate myself. I hated who I was and how I felt. And because there was no one safe to talk to, I held *everything* inside, which is a slow poisoning of the human soul.

Like most alcoholic families, mine didn't deal with problems. Because if you ever open that door, the flood comes. Where do you start and where does it end? So, you just *don't*. The belief is that what you won't acknowledge does not actually exist. But of course the monster was alive and well and slowly eating our family alive one bite at a time. To the outside world and to me, my parents, brother, and sisters appeared to be fine, so I concluded I was the only one in our family with problems.

MANAGING THE MESS

Hopeless, I began to buy into the lies in my head, further multiplying the shame and guilt. Needing to somehow numb the pain, I began to binge eat. Bill's medication of choice was booze. Mom's was an addiction to Bill. Mine became food. I would secretly go to the store and buy a stockpile of junk food—donuts, fruit pies, and various other things, all easy to eat and full of flavor with zero nutrition.

But once the bag was empty, the high was gone. Before long, eating just wasn't cutting it anymore. So I started looking for another numbing agent. Ever since I could remember, I had watched Bill turn to drinking when he was stressed out or struggling with life, so I figured alcohol might be the answer for me too. I quickly realized the big difference between food and alcohol was the enjoyment in eating is only in the moment of consumption. But booze is about what is created afterwards, and the effect is stronger and lasts much longer.

I began to drink when I was in sixth grade. At first, it was only occasional weekends. The buzz made me feel like I could conquer the world. Still very naive, I believed that no one could hurt me when I was drunk, because I no longer felt my insecurities or negative emotions. Even though they weren't really gone, they were at least covered up for a few hours and overpowered by a much better feeling. And relief of any kind was not something I had experienced much.

Every night after Bill had enough alcohol in him, his words would become increasingly sexualized and provocative. Women were objects to him, and he focused only on their looks, making comments about their bodies and how he would "love to get them in the sack." Mixed in with this bravado, he would question my mother's appearance, wanting her to wear short skirts and tight, revealing clothes. At times, he would grab her rear or breast in front of us kids. And too often, she would accommodate him.

Unfortunately, I began to absorb that interchange between my primary role models. Attention from the man and acquiescing from the woman. To get my own response from men, I decided I needed to dress in the same way and "perform" the way Bill encouraged my mom. As that belief system took form within my vulnerable, emotional state, I began to seek a response from boys to men. That is, of course, an invitation to disaster for any young lady.

All my what-ifs had brought me to the place of now asking myself, "Why *not* me?"

O Lord, how long will you forget me?

Forever?

How long will you look the other way?

How long must I struggle

with anguish in my soul,

with sorrow in my heart every day?

How long will my enemy

have the upper hand?

Turn and answer me,

O Lord my God!

Restore the sparkle to my eyes,

or I will die.

Psalm 13:1-3

CHAPTER TWO

Thirteen Going on Thirty

On my thirteenth birthday, I got all "dolled up" and went out trying to find any male willing to show me some attention—negative or otherwise. Before long, my friend and I met some guys who worked together at a retail store in our town. They asked us if we wanted to party with them. Thinking we had found what we were looking for, we said yes.

With both of us lying to our parents about where we were, we met them at a hotel room. Of course, they had plenty of alcohol on hand. Before long, I got drunk and lost all coherent thinking. Sadly, but to no one's surprise, I gave myself away to one of those guys (he had told me he was sixteen, but I later found out was twenty-one). To this day, it grieves my heart to repeat this story and wonder what must have been going on in my way-too-young-for-this mind and very immature heart.

Because of the abandonment of my birth father, the lack of approval from my adopted dad, and the wounds inflicted by the early sexual abuse, I continually searched for someone to validate my existence and fill the deep void within me. But that night in a hotel room, I discovered a new way to feel accepted and loved, even if it was only temporary, just like the junk food and alcohol abuse. Once again, I concluded that my performance was the key to getting what I wanted.

To make matters worse, my continued fantasy caused me to believe this guy must have fallen in love with me because he gave me his phone number and told me to call him. As a foolish, naive girl, I couldn't wait to call him and begin what I just knew would be our long, loving relationship. So like he said to do, the next day I called him. No answer. Later, I tried again. No answer. The next day and the next, no answer. No return calls. As the days passed and the hope of new romance faded, I got the message. Another male had used me. Another male had hurt me. Another male didn't want me. Abused. Damaged ... again.

I was so mad at myself for thinking this guy might actually like me, much less love me. For a young girl with a self-image on life support, emerging hormones, and an identity crisis, all this was too much to handle. Then add this experience to the flashbacks of the abuse and the news that Bill was not my birth father, all while being on the verge of womanhood, at least physically. With the still-open wounds cut into my heart, the pain was now beginning to create deep roots in the fertile soil of rejection and abandonment.

With regard to any healthy or supportive response from my parents, years later, I finally came to understand how they simply did not have the coping skills to deal with the extent of all I had gone through. So they did what so many do every day: sweep everything under the proverbial family rug. My growing response was to hold ever tighter to the guilt, the shame, and the fear, building a wall, brick by brick, of self-protection and self-preservation.

The destruction of my childhood innocence that began at the age of five, was now at thirteen years old sending me into a nosedive that I was starting to believe was the point of no return.

FIRST LOVE IN THE FAST LANE

With my raging hormones and rationalizations piling up, regrettably, I could not seem to stop my promiscuity. I kept believing the lie that I would somehow find acceptance if I gave boys (and I use that term intentionally) what they were looking for. Surely one of them, eventually, would love and accept me. But the vicious cycle was in motion. Fixes of temporary attention created more wounds. My warped identity caused me to assume the very next guy was going to be "the one."

But the harsh reality was frequent, shallow, and meaningless encounters. With no parental supervision, my moral compass became nonexistent as my emotional state deteriorated. While my parents didn't intentionally set out to guide their kids in the wrong direction, my mom and dad's digressing dysfunction created a horrible mess to try to navigate.

Fast-forward to my being fifteen, and I met a twenty-year-old guy named Dave. He was the nephew of one of my dad's good friends. Our families knew each other well because we had spent many weekends together while our parents partied—and we occasionally even witnessed a drunken brawl. Dave had come to our town in Montana from the Seattle area to work on his uncle's ranch. When I saw the new farmhand, it was love at first sight for me. He was handsome, well-built, fun, and more mature than the other guys I had dated. Dave and I quickly became inseparable, spending every waking hour together. After school, I would come straight home to go see him.

During this season, my parents' marital problems began to escalate. My mom discovered that my dad had been involved in an on-going affair for over two decades. Somehow he had managed to keep their time together a secret from us. After his infidelity came to light, on many nights my mom and I would drive by the "other woman's" house to see if my dad's car was there. I would watch out of the corner of my eye to see my mother's anguish or relief as we would cruise slowly past her home.

Then there were the nights when I lay awake in bed listening to my parents arguing, accusing, and assaulting each other with their verbal cuts and jabs. I constantly told my mom to leave my dad, believing that she did not deserve to be treated that way. Even as a teenager, my own insecurities and pain caused a strange empathy toward her as I watched the most important woman in my life be rejected and dismissed too. She desperately wanted to be loved and accepted just like I did. But she was being met with the same response by one man as I had experienced with many. Frustrated, I would ask her why she kept putting up with his cheating, drunkenness, and anger. Her response was always, "I have to stay for you kids."

Because of the shared pain, my mother and I decided to stick together and even began to party together. Focused on me again, Mom made me feel loved and accepted for the first time in a very long time. But our "friendship" did not allow for discipline and guidance, the very thing I truly needed as a teenager.

As my relationship with Dave deepened, my parents actually allowed him to stay in my room with me in our basement. No surprise that this lenience led to us having sex anytime we wanted. That's how caught up my parents were in their own problems. They conveniently and completely looked the other way, ignoring everything their teenage daughter was doing.

After I became an adult and then a parent, those realizations saddened me that my risky behavior was not even worth their effort to enforce any semblance of rules. But as an extremely strong-willed child, I constantly fought them tooth and nail on any authority they attempted to exert on me. What I thought was total freedom at the time, I later came to see was simply laziness and self-absorption.

With Bill's affair being discovered and his refusal to stop, my mom lost any fight she had left in her for anyone or anything. When a home is being led with immorality, why bother trying to police anyone in it? Bill likely didn't condone my actions, but he had no room to speak due to his own choices.

Because Dave was of legal age, he could buy alcohol and go to any bar whenever he wanted. With my still being underage and unable to go party with him, this allowed him to go out alone at night. He eventually started staying out for longer periods of time, obviously meeting women his own age. Then he began to not come back to our house all night. Because we were still essentially living together, I would wait up on school nights for him to come home. Ironically, my life began to reflect my mother's. When Dave would come in late, smelling of alcohol and perfume, I would put him through the same third degree I had watched my mom put Bill through: "Where have you been? Who have you been with? Do you love her? Is she more important to you than me?"

Still a teenage girl in high school but acting like a jilted wife trying to find her wayward husband, I got so desperate that I would call the bars looking for him. My confrontations made

Dave defensive and angry. One particular evening, we were at a family party. Getting more drunk as the evening went by, I became extremely disrespectful in the conversation. Eventually, after we had all gone outside, I climbed in behind the wheel of my truck but continued to loudly mouth off. Dave got so mad at me that he jumped up on the hood and, staring me down through the windshield, punched out the entire glass, shattering it into pieces inside the cab. I immediately thought he would come through the hole and hurt me, so I shut down in every way. I began to cry as Dave apologized for his angry response to my antagonizing him.

I always believed his assurances that it would never happen again, but his rage grew worse. I just kept trying to hold on to him, shooting my mouth off and adding to the distance between us. The verbal assaults soon escalated into him pushing and shoving me. Alcohol-fueled emotional and physical violence became standard behavior in our relationship.

But Dave always apologized and promised to never do it again. And my self-worth told me it was okay—a familiar yet dangerous pattern for so many women.

Guard your heart

above all else,

for it determines

the course of your life.

Proverbs 4:23

CHAPTER THREE

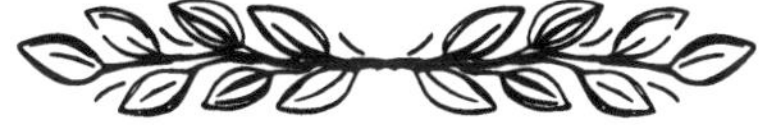

Same Song, Different Verse

As Dave and I became increasingly dysfunctional, my parents separated with both of them now focused on someone else. Their full distraction allowed me to abuse complete freedom of any authority. I would throw parties at our house for whoever wanted to join us. As the oldest sibling in our home, I was used to being the assigned caretaker of my half-sister and half-brother. But in my parents' constant absence and my selfishness, I neglected that obligation and put them in compromising situations all the time with large numbers of drunken people in our home.

I no longer kept my word with them. Anytime something came up that I deemed better than being with my siblings, I would go and leave them neglected and disappointed. But the reality was, at just fifteen years old, I was just a kid being left to parent, the last thing I was equipped to do. I was forced into being mom and dad when I wasn't even able to take care of myself. Regrettably, I deeply hurt my sister and brother with my actions during that time of our lives.

Like so many teenagers, I was extremely self-consumed. I thought the world revolved around me. Yet somehow in all the craziness, Dave and I managed to stick together over the next few years. Following my high school graduation, we decided to move into his parents' home in the Seattle area. We both found jobs, and I sincerely believed the new scenery would help our relationship. I desperately wanted less drinking and no other women, and therefore no fights.

I thought I could keep a tight rein on Dave in his family's home. In a relationship built on damage and deceit, my insecurities and lack of trust caused me to question him most of the time. But Dave was always wonderful with words, and he would tell me, "Tonya, no more women or alcohol. I promise." He would assure me I was the "only one" for him.

One night, seemingly out of the blue, Dave asked me to marry him. To his and my surprise, I answered, "One day I'll say yes, but not yet." While I loved him dearly, something inside me knew I could not keep living in such tumult. And as our fighting continued to escalate, one night during a war of words, he punched me in the face. Somehow, my tooth cut into my cheek and caused a scar that is still there to this day. That alone should have shown me it was time to get out of this toxic situation. But Dave was so guilt-ridden for hitting me that he bought me a promise ring as a peace offering. Helplessly hopeful, I saw this gesture as a positive sign of change and acceptance. I took the ring and put it on my finger, agreeing to marry him someday.

There was always a faint voice deep in my soul that would whisper, "You deserve better." But as so many women falsely perceive about "their men," a fantasy world conjures a belief that the right woman can change the wrong man. My performance-minded determination convinced me I could not give up and I had to make this relationship work, even if it killed one of us. How many of us ladies have had this belief hold us captive for far too long?

Around this same time, I met Judy, an older woman who worked next door to where I did, and we developed a friendship. She became a sort of mother figure to me, as she listened to my struggles with Dave and offered me encouragement. She invited me to church, and I went a couple of times with her, although the sermons I heard there fell mostly on deaf ears. After some time, Judy began to encourage me to leave Dave and go back to school to get my degree. She saw a potential in me that no one had ever expressed to me before.

Judy's advice eventually mustered up enough of my courage that I left Dave. I was determined to make the changes that had eluded me time and time again. Once free from the relationship, I moved back to Montana, enrolled in a local university, and started classes. But just changing scenery without changing the heart usually leads us right back to the same places. I really enjoyed college life, but I continued to feed my need for affirmation by allowing myself to be used by men. When I would go out with girlfriends, I sometimes consumed so much alcohol that I would black out. On occasion, I would wake up not fully knowing how I got where I was and what I had done.

One time after I drank and blacked out at a frat party, the next morning I couldn't remember much about the night before. However, my college roommates made sure I knew all the indecency I had engaged in. Embarrassment and shame overwhelmed me. They all begged me to not drink so much. My behavior made them uncomfortable, and they likely also felt responsible for protecting me from myself first and guys second. But like I had done so many times before, I ignored their warnings and pleas and every single red flag that had been waved in my face. I dismissed reality and kept on partying.

A MATTER OF LIFE AND DEATH

Dave began calling, trying to get back together with me. And I did miss him. On one call he asked to come visit me. I decided this would be my chance to really help this guy and change him. *Ironic, right? Delusional even?* When Dave picked me up, we went dancing and drinking. For the first time in longer than I could recall, we didn't fight and actually had a great time. I was ecstatic because I truly thought we could turn the page and start a new chapter together.

Grateful for a great night, Dave wanted to get right back into our relationship. While I agreed, I gave him a long list of conditions—in other words, what he would have to do to make it work this time. The big three were no getting drunk, no other women, and coming home at a decent hour. Promising he was now a new man, he pledged his love for me and proclaimed he would never lose me again. He willingly agreed to all my rules, so we gave romance another chance.

Being in two different cities at this point, we talked on the phone often. One weekend I decided to surprise him with a visit. After driving eight hours one way, when I got to his house he was obviously getting dressed to go out. I was shocked. While he was in the bathroom, I got his phone and simply hit redial. After the first ring, a young female voice gave me an excited hi, obviously thinking it was Dave.

Furious, I confronted her, asking who she was and how she knew my boyfriend. Surprised and defensive, she stated that *she* was his girlfriend and they had been dating exclusively for a couple of months. I could not believe this was happening to me again. Another man was deceiving me. Except this time was the second go-round!

I hung up on the now just-as-stunned-and-angry-as-me girl, stormed into the bathroom, and began screaming and yelling profanities at Dave. I obviously knew *what* was happening again, but this time I demanded to hear some kind of *why*.

Enraged at him but furious with myself for falling prey again, I took off the promise ring he gave me, cocked my arm back like a major league pitcher, and threw it at him full force at close range. Crying hysterically, the last thing I said to him on my way out the door was, "You are a loser and a psychotic jerk! I never want to see you again—ever!" I put just as much force into slamming his front door as I had into throwing his ring at him.

Dave had taken my heart, ripped it to pieces, and walked on what little was left of me. As much as I could understand love at my young age and maturity, I sincerely had deep feelings for him and believed I wanted to be with him for the rest of my life.

One month later, almost to the day, after I had walked out on Dave after having the last word, I received a phone call. He had committed suicide by shooting himself at his parents' home. All he left behind was a note … to me.

The letter began by telling me how he had tried to get in touch with me, but of course I had never answered his calls. He went on to tell me how much he loved me and never meant to hurt me. He asked that I would always remember him in my dreams.

As you might imagine, guilt ripped through me. I thought, *I'm to blame. I caused his death. I may as well have been the one to pull the trigger.* Following the barrage of accusations, the horrible what-ifs began. *What if I had taken his call? What if I had forgiven him? Would he still be alive? Could I have stopped this from happening?*

This was my doing. He all but said so in his letter. I could have been the one to save him. But I had failed at it all—I couldn't get him to quit drinking or quit other women, I couldn't keep him home, and now I couldn't even keep him alive. One conclusion now bookended with what happened to me at five years old: *This must be my fault. I'm a failure. Always have been.*

Yet again, my identity was being defined by the wounds created from bad decisions and choices driven by just wanting love, acceptance, and approval. Every time I thought I had no room left for more pain, I was sadly mistaken. The smothering layers kept coming, piling on one by one, with shame and guilt creating callouses on my heart, weighing down my soul. That much pain has a strange, ironic effect after a while: you start to get numb. And numbness means you start to feel *nothing* at all.

After a short season of trying desperately to climb out of where I had been and fight my way up to a new place I had never been before, the nightmare ending with Dave's death sent me into a tailspin.

You have kept record
of my days of wandering.
You have stored my tears
in your bottle
and counted each of them.

Psalm 56:8 CEV

CHAPTER FOUR

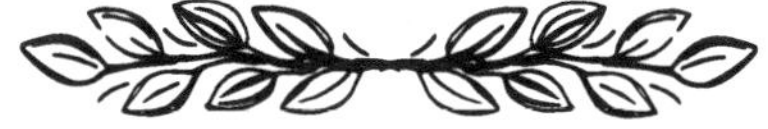

Alcohol, Anger, and an Ultimatum

Dave's suicide took me to the darkest place I had ever been. So I turned to the two things I knew best: bars and the guys in them. To say I was out of control was a gross understatement. I wanted to either feel good or feel nothing. Those were the only options I would accept.

For a while I tried to stay focused on college, but my emotional state finally forced me to take a break. Back in my original bad environment, the destruction continued, bar to bar and encounter to encounter.

Soon my former employer reached out and asked me to come back to work there, and once again feeling the pull on my gypsy soul, I decided to move back to the Seattle area. My dear friend, Judy, offered for me to live with her family. With her as my support system, I thought this would be a good opportunity to begin to work through my issues. Once again, she shared her faith with me and offered a different path, but I just couldn't fathom any source of love and grace, human or otherwise.

Working full-time again provided a new outlet, but the loneliness of being so far from home was much harder this time. Added to that were the memories and reminders of Dave that seemed to be everywhere, which circled me right back to my pain and poor decisions. Trying to run from something I could never escape, going back and forth between Montana and Washington, I moved back home yet again.

Back with my old friends on one particular night, I was partying with them and, of course, blacked out. But this time they all left me. The next morning, I woke up completely disoriented, next to someone I didn't know. Lying there in my fogged thoughts, attempting to piece anything together of the night before, I became concerned and afraid. *How did this happen? Who is this guy? Did I somehow consent or was I raped?*

As I processed the situation, regardless of my drunken state, I blamed the guy for what he had obviously done, and I considered it rape. But the struggle within me was that I had been the one who intentionally decided to drink until I blacked out. As I so often did, my mind went back to when I was a little girl. If my parents didn't take abuse and violence seriously, why should anyone believe me now when I had passed out? My behavior was always the unknown variable when I woke up the next morning. But this time was different. I felt like the outcome was clear. Alcohol never failed me, always doing its job to make me forget. But add bars and bad boys to the equation and the result was another disaster.

Every time I thought I had maxed out the amount of guilt and shame I could possibly feel, I found a new low. For the first time in my young life, I stopped looking at everyone else and started questioning what was wrong with *me*. I faced the harsh reality that I was self-destructive, not just occasionally but all the time.

As humans, when we are in considerable pain, particularly emotional pain, we run to something. Once there, we try to hide. What was Adam and Eve's first response when they realized in the garden that they had disobeyed God? They ran and hid. But hiding from God didn't work then and it still doesn't. Yet we run and hide, even when we know the destination is bad for us.

The world is full of hiding places for sinners. But *none* of them are safe. *None* of them are secure. They all ultimately expose us in our nakedness before a holy God. I was no different. I spent my days working, my nights and weekends running, and trying desperately to hide. But the wounds so heavily inflicted on my heart were now making me realize I had gone from a victim of others to a victim of myself. I wasted so many years, too many years, in the vicious cycle of downward spiral.

Brick by brick, I had constructed an emotional wall that wouldn't allow anyone access to me, most especially with men. They might abuse me, but they would never get through to who I truly was. I would not allow that kind of intimacy. I would protect myself at all cost. Like anyone living wounded, I had a perception of reality that was distorted and destructive, not protective. Filled with despair, I had completely run out of *any* hope. I came to the conclusion that I wanted to die. I had no purpose. I was sure of that

As my new self-realizations kept coming, I stumbled across an overriding, dominant emotion—anger. I. Was. Angry! Even though it probably wasn't always visible on the outside, I was filled with rage. I lived in a bitter state about *everything* that had happened in my life. Sexual abuse, physical abuse, verbal abuse, emotional abuse, all leading to my new title: I was a drunk. Something I never wanted to be. My experiences in life had shaped my thinking. My thinking had not shaped my experiences.

A SOBERING THOUGHT

One night I was at a local bar, consuming shots and on the verge of another blackout. Somehow, before I hit the wall, I managed to stumble across the street to a friend's house. I threw myself on his couch and passed out. A couple of hours later, his roommate, Rich, came home from working a night shift. The door opening and closing woke me from my stupor, and I was coherent enough to talk.

I felt an immediate connection to this guy, but I was sure it was no different from any other time. But Rich *was* different—not at all like the other now nameless, faceless guys I had met over the years. He opened up and shared about his own challenges with alcohol and told me that he had made the decision to stop drinking. A man confessing change and sobriety was not something I had encountered before! Drawn to him in a very different way, when I asked about us going out sometime, he agreed.

I decided it would be a nice change of pace to invite him over for a homecooked meal. That evening, we talked for hours. There was definitely chemistry between us, so senselessly, we got physical. However, the big difference was that Rich was somehow able to break through my wall of protection, and a deep-rooted emotional bond quickly formed.

I liked how Rich handled himself as a well-put-together man. He didn't party. He was a gentleman around women. He even opened doors for me. But he was just coming out of a relationship, so he was not so quick to embrace dating. He told me he wanted to take things slowly and let it progress gradually. Yet each time we got together became physical. That, of course, is not slow and gradual.

As we kept seeing one another, Rich began to question my drinking. I was always quick to justify myself and refused to acknowledge a problem. To make matters worse, I had taken a job as a bartender, so sobriety was a farfetched concept to me. If I admitted to anyone, much less Rich, that I was an alcoholic, then I would also have to admit I was my worst nightmare: a drunk.

In an attempt to take steps to address my past, I started to see a female counselor. I talked to her about Rich's concerns, and she gave me a quick "see if you might have a drinking problem" test. There were ten questions and if I answered more than five with yes, then I likely had a problem. Being honest, I answered yes to all ten.

So it was official. I definitely had a problem. But my response to the test and the outcome? I left the counselor's office and got drunk!

Regardless of the blackouts or number of shots or twelve-packs of beer in a night, I came to the conclusion that I just needed to "cut back a little." Alcoholics are always looking to escape reality, and I was not ready to face reality of any kind—because everything I had dreaded was now coming true. I had become my parents. I was repeating the cycle, dealing with life just like I had witnessed growing up. I tried to hide my drinking from Rich, but to no avail.

I decided that if I visited the local rehab center, they would be able to show me how to be a "controlled drinker." So I set up an appointment and took my mom with me for moral support. I assumed they would tell me how to be less obnoxious and how to stop before a blackout. Following a lengthy interview, I took all their psychoanalytic tests. Afterwards, they sat my mom and me down at a huge conference table and had the audacity to tell me I was much sicker than I thought. They advised me to check into their facility and agree to confinement for the full twenty-eight days!

All my theories were now blown out of the water, and I immediately regretted my decision to walk into this place. They had just confirmed that I was indeed a drunk. Evidently, at a twenty-eight-day-confinement level, the worst kind. My wounds *were* defining my life.

Telling them I needed to think about it, which I'm sure they heard a lot as an excuse to get out the door and never come back, my mom and I left. But I took their information with me. All the way home, I dreaded telling Rich that they agreed with him and he was right.

LINE IN THE SAND

That night, when I shared with Rich the treatment center's "crazy analysis" of my problem, he said something I will never forget: "Well, Tonya, if you want to continue a relationship with me, I need you to get sober. If you can't, this is over. . . . End of story."

After dating for six months and enduring my insane alcohol abuse, Rich was not willing to proceed any further in the relationship if I refused to change. His sobriety was important to him, and under no circumstances was he going to chance losing all he had worked so hard to obtain because of some tanked-up girl. His feelings for me couldn't jeopardize his health and future. Rich took a stand, and I could tell he was not going to back down.

All I was ever used to a guy ultimately wanting out of a relationship was sex, so I was shocked by his concern for me and his confidence in his decision. I decided to listen to him. Because I liked Rich. He was different. There was something distinctive about him. And the biggest draw of them all: he had captured my heart.

I finally gave in and gave up. Waved the white flag. Agreed to treatment. Twenty-eight days to sift through *years* of wounds and lies. And the thought of struggling through all of it was overwhelming, to say the least.

The end of a matter
is better than its beginning,
and patience
is better than pride.

Ecclesiastes 7:8 NIV

CHAPTER FIVE

Realizations and Revelations

I checked in for my twenty-eight-day journey toward healing, and began the arduous processing of every experience, emotion, and pain, all to be faced head-on with no numbing agents. One issue that quickly festered to the top was quite clear: I absolutely hated men. Capital H. *All* men. In the intense agony of my confession sessions, I emotionally threw up all my years of testosterone-induced nausea, how every guy I had ever met had wronged me, hurt me, and/or abused me. And, in the end, always left me disappointed, disillusioned, and emotionally disfigured.

No man had *ever* protected *me*. No man had ever provided for me. None of them had done what we are told real men are *supposed* to do. As far as I was concerned, they had *all* forsaken their God-given duty. I arrived at the conclusion that I was a failure because every man in my life had failed me. All their sins, mistakes, and selfishness had created the mess I had become. The symptom that drove me to rehab may have been alcohol, but to me, the real source of the sickness was men.

I made up my mind that the entire gender was ignorant, inept, insensitive, and self-seeking. All were fools who only wanted *one thing* from a woman. They all used women to fulfill their own self-focused sexual desires and, in turn, create an atmosphere of power and control so they can keep getting what they want. These deep, intense feelings led me to a constant state of self-protection and self-preservation.

My confessions in rehab led to a burning question in my heart and my spirit: Was there—is there—a man out there, somewhere, anywhere, who won't fail me, won't hurt me, who will protect and provide for me? Maybe even rescue me from all this pain and heal my wounds? By the end of my first week of rehab, I was more convinced than ever that answer was an unfortunate no.

Through my counseling, I began to realize that wounded people work hard to never come across as vulnerable. The lie is that you will then become an easy target for harm. The collective culture of our modern world is all about power and the accumulation of things, which translates to a fully driven performance-based society. For these reasons, many people view *any* sign of vulnerability as true weakness. That was most certainly my worldview.

Too often I was told, "You just need to buck up. Toughen up, girl." In my circles, if you were weak, you would be eaten alive. This pattern of thinking defined who I became. I was a woman with something to prove. I carried a big chip on my shoulder, waiting for someone to act as if they might try to knock it off. That attitude was a façade for the wounds of abandonment, rejection, shame, and guilt.

Those were some of the realizations that came to me through counseling and treatment that began to lay a foundation toward change. I did well in rehab and graduated from treatment in December 1994, and Rich and I got married in July 1995. In between rehab and our wedding, I became pregnant with our first child, but sadly, I miscarried.

As with all people who have experienced that specific loss and pain, the trauma was very difficult for me to process and deal with. Working to apply all the tools I had been given to stay sober during this grief was challenging. But I was able to get pregnant again, and our baby was born in January 1996.

To sum up the Tonya timeline, I got sober, got pregnant, miscarried, married, got pregnant again, and had a baby. Through all the ups and downs, I somehow managed to stay away from alcohol. But I still couldn't escape the constant wounds of life.

WAKING NIGHTMARE

My mom and Bill's pattern over the years went back and forth from trying their relationship again to separation. In August 1997, a time they were back together, I received a frantic call from my dad to come to their home right away. Bill never called me, so I knew something was very wrong. Beside myself, I jumped into my car and raced to their house. I cried out to God, begging, "Please, no! Not my mom! Don't let this be about my mom! Don't take her from me!"

I flew into the driveway and ran inside to find Bill sitting on the stairs with his face in his hands, sobbing. "What's wrong?!" I blurted out.

He looked up and said through his tears, "Your mom, Tonya … she's gone."

Feeling like an unseen force punched me in the gut, I doubled over and fell to my knees. "No! Not my mom! No! No!" I cried. Crumpling all the way to the floor in tears, I screamed, "No! This can't be!"

My mom and I were at a good place. Once again best friends, we talked every day. I could not understand why she had been taken from me so suddenly. I went from sobbing to feeling like I couldn't breathe. The overwhelming sense of loss and loneliness was too much to bear. And all the questions flew through my mind. *Who will ever love me like my mom? Who could ever love me like that? Who will make me feel like everything will be okay when it isn't?*

Suddenly, I flashbacked to a haunting nightmare I'd had. I had dreamed that my mom would die in a motorcycle accident. Following that, I constantly reminded her to wear her helmet. She would strap it to the bike every time she rode, but rarely wore it. I always nagged her about riding safety.

But my mom died from trauma in a tragic motorcycle accident. She was not wearing her helmet.

I wondered, *What if she had listened to me? Would she still be alive?* My negative thought patterns kicked in and guilt set in—again. First Dave, then the miscarriage, and now my mom. Another life I loved, lost. Gone too soon. Another person I had failed to save. But the loss of my mother was like nothing I had ever experienced before. All the while, I was working so hard to stay sober.

TORTUOUS TIMING

Not long before my mom died, Rich and I had both lost our jobs due to "corporate downsizing." We had a newborn baby and no clear career path, so when Rich was offered a position in Charlotte, North Carolina, we felt we had no choice but to go. In just three days, we were scheduled to move two thousand miles cross-country.

My younger sister and brother were still at home with Bill, and I did not want to leave them at such a horrible time in all our lives. My family needed me and I needed them. Mom had always been the glue for our dysfunctional bunch, so who would hold the family together now? She had been the cheerleader for us all, and now everyone was at their lowest point.

I felt like if I left my sister and brother now, I would be abandoning them. First losing their mom, and then just days later, their sister too. Reluctant as I was, however, I knew I had to go and begin my new life with my husband and baby. One of my most familiar emotions, guilt from creating disappointment, had me by the heart. I perceived my life as one big letdown to those around me. Leaving my family at the worst possible time was yet another milestone in the mess.

While Rich was understanding and supportive, he knew we couldn't stay in Montana. As hard as the decision was, we left and began our long journey. While driving through the switchbacks of Durango, Colorado, I told Rich that I had an odd sense that our move to Charlotte was about more than financial security. I felt it was about something so much bigger than an income. I couldn't quite discern what, but *something* was waiting for us there.

REACHING OUT, LOOKING UP

Losing my mom was the most difficult thing I had ever endured. Her death had broken my heart. The bright future I thought was ahead for my new family now had a dark shadow cast over it because of the tragedy in my birth family.

I wondered how long it might be, if ever, before any light of hope would shine in my wounded soul.

In the moments around my mom's death and other tragedies that came into my life, I prayed 9-1-1 prayers. I had heard of God and about Heaven enough to cry out for any sort of help from whoever might be listening. But I had never read a page of the Bible and had only gone to church a couple of times with Judy. She had given me a Bible. For the first few years, I kept it close by but never actually opened it. And then my mom's death sent me on a search for something different to ease my pain. I knew I couldn't drink. I would not go back to that crazy lifestyle, and I knew that if I ever did, that would be the end of me. But with such a deep feeling of hopelessness, I desperately wanted to numb the pain. Yet maybe this time I might find something positive, actually helpful?

After we got settled in Charlotte, Rich said he believed we needed to attend church as a family. I had no idea what we were looking for, but I figured that if it would help our marriage and my wounds, it was worth a try. My old habits weren't really working for me anymore, and the desire to seek "something more" now overwhelmed my heart. As I longed to fill the void in my soul, we began visiting churches of all styles, flavors, and sizes. They don't call the Southeast the Bible Belt for nothing. There are a lot, like *a lot,* of churches.

Even after visiting four churches, we hadn't felt a connection anywhere. Then I came across a Christian radio station and decided to call them to ask for a recommendation. I innocently was unaware of whatever the special formula was to pick a church, but the radio announcer kindly invited us to visit the one he attended: Hickory Grove Baptist Church. I thought, *Why not?*

Although the church was huge, Dr. Joe Brown preached with boldness about the saving grace of a God who offered hope and healing. Hope *and* healing—that sounded way too good to be true. That night after our first visit to Hickory Grove, two gentlemen who attended there came by to invite us to their Sunday school class. They also invited me to a ladies' Bible study. Now, when I thought of a "ladies' Bible study," I imagined little old ladies sitting around drinking tea and constantly using words like *thee* and *thou* with an occasional fire-and-brimstone reference thrown in.

I decided to go anyway, and found it to be quite the contrary. The ladies were just finishing up a lesson on loving their husbands—and they were even talking about sex. I could not believe my ears! These were not little old prudes. They were digging into the details of their marriages. I immediately thought that if they only knew what I was going through or who I really was, they would never want me to come back.

During our church search, I continued to live in a secret battle with depression, feeling lost and unloved, and missing my mom terribly. I was lifeless, spending days lying around the house, barely summoning the emotional strength to take care of our daughter. I could not escape the black cloud of depression hanging over my life.

Rich encouraged me to get some help, and taking his advice, I visited a psychiatrist who put me on medication. *Lots* of medication. He diagnosed me with PTSD—post-traumatic stress disorder—and also depression and anxiety. I had a different drug for each condition. Now I was legally medicated and numbed in a socially acceptable way from a doctor, but at least this regimen helped me survive the darkness and stay alive each day.

Rich and I continued to visit the new church. On one particular Sunday, while we were feeling especially broken and hopeless, with no notice at all, the Spirit moved in our hearts. Something different came over us, and we gave our lives to Christ. We were then baptized together. I really want to tell you that I had this immediate, miraculous sense of power and my life changed overnight. I'd like to, but that would be a lie.

Even so, Christ's love for us was being birthed in our hearts. While I had searched so many times in so many ways to find something, anything, anyone to change me, this time, something, Someone found *me*. And then I remembered the big question that had come out of my revelation in rehab. Maybe there was a Man out there who wouldn't fail me and wouldn't hurt me, who would protect and provide for me? One who would rescue me from all my pain and heal my wounds?

Hope. For the first time in my life, I began to experience hope.

And this hope will not lead to disappointment.
For we know how dearly God loves us,
because he has given us the Holy Spirit
to fill our hearts with his love.
When we were utterly helpless,
Christ came at just the right time
and died for us sinners.

Romans 5:5–6

CHAPTER SIX

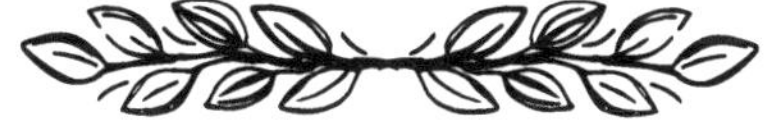

Facing Myself, Finding Family, Following Jesus

With Rich's job established in Charlotte and after several failed attempts for me to find a job, we decided I would stay home to care for our daughter and our home. This was foreign to me because I had always worked an outside job and had strong feelings about helping to provide for my family. Dealing with my mom's sudden death and being so far away from home, I was extremely lonely. Rich's family members were the only connections I had there, so I took a step of faith and began reaching out to the ladies of the church Bible study. I also began attending local AA meetings.

With the women at church, I had no problem staying on a surface level because I struggled to let them in further. My marriage to Rich was shaky because I had so many wounds. I didn't even know where to start to work through my issues. I wanted no one to know the truth about my PTSD and depression. I thought a lot about my past—alcohol, food, drugs, sex, money, pride, people-pleasing, and the quick-fix appeal they offered. Yet in the end, I knew they were all like putting a band-aid on a gunshot wound.

My newfound faith in Christ helped me see that I did not want to pass down my wounds to my daughter. The last thing I wanted was for her to learn to live life defined by wounds. I saw how Jesus was working in my church family, my friend Judy, and even in Rich, but I was still struggling. I knew I needed what they were experiencing. I wanted what I saw in them, but still battled on a daily basis with the will to live. I believed my options were limited, and I struggled to escape darkness and despair.

Eventually, one day at a time, sometimes one moment at a time, God got my attention. He began to break through my hardened fortress and show me how He could take over and define my life. Even though I had prayed that morning with the pastor and Rich in the church service and we were baptized, I knew I had to make the choice to place *all* of my trust in Christ. I had to let go of everything I had held on to for far too long. And then I had to grab hold of Him to rescue me from sin and lies and anger and pain. Ultimately, He had to rescue me from *myself*.

Then and now, my faith journey is a *daily* decision. Even on the best days, this choice to follow Christ is extremely difficult. He never said it would be easy. In fact, if you read the Gospels, Jesus makes it quite clear that the path to Him is narrow. Not because of Him, but rather the constant encroachment of the Enemy and the world.

I was a wounded woman who had *never* been able to trust anyone except my mother, and she was gone. And yet here I was, making the decision to put my complete trust in Someone I could not even see! If you have never experienced this draw to faith, I know that sounds crazy. I was skeptical too. At that time in my life, *knowing* something and *believing* something were two very different things, but the ladies in the Bible study and the folks in our Sunday school class loved my family like nothing I had ever experienced from anyone. Receiving unconditional love is like sitting a beggar down at a banquet table. The food may be *available*, but the *access* is hard to fathom.

When our first Christmas in Charlotte came around, we didn't have much. One Saturday morning while Rich was at work, someone knocked at our door. When I opened it, all the people from our Sunday school class were standing there. They started singing Christmas carols as they handed over armloads of gifts for us—a Christmas tree, decorations, furniture, toys, food, and money.

As I witnessed this amazing expression and explosion of love, the only response I could manage was to weep. I wondered why on earth these people would do this. So I asked them and they answered with, "Because God is good." Ironically, I had no idea what that meant. I didn't understand such a response. But then one of them said, "This is just what you do for your family." I thought, *What family? I'm not related to any of them.* After they left, we had more presents under our tree than I had ever seen. When Rich got home from work, he was as speechless as I was.

What I finally came to realize about that day was once you become a member of God's family, you are *never* fatherless, motherless, or alone. You are an orphan no more. All those years of feeling like I was not acceptable or loved were changing through what I experienced from these people. God knew I needed to experience this kind of love, and my life was now being changed—and I would continue to be transformed forever.

Over the next five years, these families continued to offer love, care, and counsel, as well as emotional and financial support to us. Motivated by the love and grace of Christ, they took us in and grew us up in their family. I had always thought love had to have strings attached. Never had I seen unselfish, unconditional love from others. Maybe from my mom, but never from people I barely knew.

I had lived most of my life operating out of a wounded spirit that wreaked havoc on my family and my belief system. God had to show me I was going about life all wrong. I was not building others up; I was tearing them down. Living out of fear, I spent so much time directing my anger in the wrong place, rather than dealing with the pain. That lifestyle led to my hurting others.

I finally came to a crossroads while working through my wounds: I had to decide if I would live in Hell here on earth, always wondering why God would allow such things, while also doubting His goodness, or choose to believe that He is good and has a plan for my pain. And I came to see that my pain is a part of His story to define who I am and who I have become.

SURRENDER TO FREEDOM

My very personal and intimate story, I believe, makes it crystal clear that I tried the world's way one-hundred percent, head-on, full tilt. I spent so many years trying to cover up abandonment, physical abuse, sexual abuse, loneliness, suicidal thoughts, loss of loved ones, miscarriages, financial ruin, loss of jobs, family conflict, and severe depression and anxiety. *Nothing* I tried worked to heal the pain associated with those wounds, including the daily attempts to numb my pain with alcohol, drugs, sex, money, food, power, manipulation, pride, silence, control, and anger.

In my most desperate state, to try to salvage some sort of life, I took what I felt at the time was my last option: I surrendered my life to Jesus Christ. I decided to not live for myself anymore, but to live for Him. I can tell you from firsthand experience that He is the only reason my life was saved.

The reality is we are all flawed humans, afraid to surrender because we fear giving up control. But that is a lie. Submission and surrender are not about giving up anything; they are actually about freedom. Our rebellion against God causes us to be like a powerful locomotive that looks over as it runs seventy miles an hour down the tracks and longs to be on the open road, free to go anywhere it wants. But a train without tracks can go nowhere. It is effectively stuck, grounded. Surrendering to who God created us to be, running on His tracks, is the *only* true freedom in this world.

I finally realized that my shame and guilt had me in an emotional and spiritual prison with no hope of pardon. Toxic emotions ruled my thoughts and actions. If you have ever suffered from anxiety attacks, you know the feeling of being so anxious that you cannot breathe, and no matter how many deep breaths you try to take, it still feels like someone is sitting on your chest. The insanity of living in that state is overwhelming. But a personal relationship with Christ can free you from all the tumult and toxicity, allowing you the freedom to truly breathe … and live.

We were created for a purpose by a Master Planner. A life full of hope and purpose is available to you too. A life of freedom is waiting for you. The legacy you are creating and will pass on to your kids can be one of meaning and blessing for generations to come.

YOUR TURN, YOUR TIME

I hope you can see how my introduction to Jesus Christ changed everything and began to transform my life through healing and hope. The great news is that God offers this opportunity to anyone. Acts 2:21 is clear, "But everyone who calls on the name of the Lord will be saved."

If you related to any or all of my story and are in a place where you have little hope and life seems to be digging a deeper pit for you, I want to share with you the hope in Christ that can free you.

I have participated in many of the ways of the world that promised satisfaction and "the good life." However, nothing could be further from the truth. The ways of the world can look so enticing on the front end, but ultimately, when you are wounded, you keep looking for comfort in any possible scenario. Yet, those will always, and I mean *always,* take you further than you intended and will leave you emptier than you ever anticipated.

The reality is that people and things will always disappoint us, but God *never* will. I promise you that a life surrendered to Christ is full of hope, courage, and authentic legacy. A life apart from Him is marked by pain with no hope or meaning. If you know you need help to work through the pain that has you operating out of a wounded spirit, I want to encourage you to surrender your life to Christ, just as I did. Take a moment to pray with a humble heart and acknowledge you are a sinner, meaning you have gone your own way and have disobeyed God. Tell Him you are ready to live a changed life. Surrender your will to the Lord and then begin to follow His ways.

God gives you the choice. If you are ready to begin a relationship with Christ, there is a strong likelihood that someone in your life would love to know, and is ready to talk with you about this important choice and answer any questions to guide you in your decision. Please talk to a Christian friend or family member as soon as you can.

If you know you are ready to begin a relationship with Christ right now, while there are no magic words or a specific formula for receiving God's gift of salvation, here is a simple prayer for guidance:

"Dear God, I know I am a sinner and need Your forgiveness. I now turn from my sins and ask You into my life to be my Savior and Lord. I choose to follow You, Jesus. Please forgive my sins and give me Your gift of eternal life. Thank You for dying for me, saving me, and changing my life. In Jesus' name, amen."

For I am not ashamed
of this Good News about Christ.
It is the power of God at work,
saving everyone who believes.

Romans 1:16

CHAPTER SEVEN

Decide to No Longer Be a Victim

I have told you about my journey to faith in Jesus Christ, and at the end of the previous chapter, I invited you to make the same decision I did. If you have already trusted Christ, or if you did so at that point in the book, now I want to get into some truths I have learned in my own maturity and healing. If you still aren't sure about this "Jesus thing," I understand. As I told you, I struggled for a while with faith and trust too. Should you make the decision to take God up on His offer, you can go back to that spot in the book anytime. Until you take your last breath, you can make the choice for Him.

For so many of us, the source of our wounds has been someone hurting us, so we decide no one can be trusted. But trust is essential to a relationship with Jesus Christ, who can transform our lives. Trusting in the healing power of Christ displays emotional and spiritual maturity as well as intelligence. This is found only in the power of Christ's sacrifice for us on the cross and His resurrection. Yet, transformation can occur only if we choose to overcome our past and trust Him. He offers salvation, but He will never force Himself on anyone.

Everyone's story of how they became wounded is different. Even so, the end result is often the same. Many plummet into a cycle of perfectionism, driven to "try harder" and adopting a performance mindset, just like I did. Others hide behind a disguise of lies, isolation, and emotional brick walls, also what I did.

I now want to share some deeper truths I have learned and am still working on daily. Once we make the choice to no longer be a victim of anyone or any circumstance, how do we experience real freedom from all the wounds and negative feelings and behaviors?

When a cut on the body is deep and becomes infected, we cannot leave it unattended for long. Even a relatively small cut can potentially create a life-threatening situation. We have to go to a physician to have it cleaned and bandaged, and then take an antibiotic to prevent or stop infection. For the wounds to our hearts and souls, we need a Great Physician to heal us. In Mark 2, Jesus used a medical analogy to explain why He chose to hang out with "sinners" over the religious leaders of the day.

> *Later, Levi invited Jesus and his disciples to his home as dinner guests, along with many tax collectors and other disreputable sinners. (There were many people of this kind among Jesus' followers.) But when the teachers of religious law who were Pharisees saw him eating with tax collectors and other sinners, they asked his disciples, "Why does he eat with such scum?" When Jesus heard this, he told them, "Healthy people don't need a doctor—sick people do. I have come to call not those who think they are righteous, but those who know they are sinners" (Mark 2:15–17).*

THE ILLUSION OF CONTROL

For many years I lived in a condition where I was determined to take back what had been taken from me or to regain control of what I had lost control of. Control meant two things: no one could hurt me again, and nothing bad could happen to me again. But what I had not yet learned was that the desire for control is just the byproduct of fear and distrust. Attempting to control others' behavior was really all about me, to try to force things to turn out the way I wanted so I could avoid any unpleasant emotions.

The desire to control is typically present for one or more of the following reasons:

- Victim mindset
- Fear of the outcome
- Pride/ego
- Power trip/control
- Distrust
- Self-protection
- To avoid an appearance of weakness or vulnerability
- Selfishness/self-centeredness

Any effort to control emotions, individuals, and/or environments by our behavior is often attempted by manipulation, anger, bargaining, silence, feigned kindness, backstabbing, lying, and so on. In my case, I thought I had power and was in control of my situation. However, all I really had was an adrenaline high from trying to constantly create the *illusion* of an atmosphere of control.

What I was actually doing was destroying the relationships around me by committing to the daunting task of 24/7/365 construction of "The Great Wall of Tonya." I was determined that nothing and no one would get through to me, no matter the cost. Yet this just furthered my efforts of self-protection as I tried to prove that women are superior and men are inept. So many wounded women like I was end up trying to escape more hurt, searching for identity and looking for a purpose they cannot find, which leads to a life of self-indulgence, compromised relationships, promiscuity, drugs, self-protection, and feelings of bitterness and rage.

I determined the best way to cope with all these wrongs was to foster a mindset of victimization, which allowed me a false sense of security that kept me entrapped in my wounds. I chose to hide behind self-justified bad behaviors. I believed if I trusted anyone, they would try to capitalize on my vulnerability, and I was not going to allow that. If you can relate to my story, then it's likely that a person of authority wounded you somewhere along the way, and a belief system of distrust became rooted in your being.

If all our responses to life are based on our wounds and the lies that have been embedded into our hearts, then we are defined by those wounds. Wounded people most often have an inaccurate view of reality. Unhealed hurts force us into self-protection mode. We develop a false belief that if we rely on ourselves to control, manipulate, lie, and fake it, then we will not have to worry about more pain. We believe we know how to take care of ourselves and we can run our own show.

Self-protection appealed to me because, by my own estimation, every man in my life had not protected me and had left me with significant wounds. Thus, I continued on the destructive path of keeping everyone at arm's length, never really allowing others to get to know me. For years, I even refused to let my husband Rich know me intimately, because I was so fearful of more rejection or abandonment.

Believing we can control our own lives creates a false sense of power, providing a constant distraction from the real, deep-rooted issues. If we are engaged in a belief system that we are in control, we will be dreadfully crushed when something happens that our beliefs cannot explain.

When the inevitable comes, we fight back harder each time, believing we were supposed to control what happened to us. That is what happened to me with the deaths of both Dave and my mother.

Trying to control a desirable outcome over which we have no power can hurt us deeply as women, and, in turn, detrimentally affect our families and ultimately society as a whole. Believing we can live predictable lives is a lie, because bad things will happen that are beyond what we can regulate. And, in the end, we are only responsible for our attitude and actions in response to situations that are out of our control.

If you look at why people attempt to control their environments, you will always find fear—fear of getting hurt again, fear of incompetency, fear of disappointment, and/or fear of failure. The greater the fear, the greater the desire to control all possible outcomes. But what can we actually control? Not much. For those who struggle with this issue, not all come across as outwardly controlling. Many try to control with cold and unloving silence, which is just as detrimental to relationships as an environment of outspoken resistance. Regardless of the approach, this is based on fear followed by learned behavior.

The lies we as women are led to believe need to be rejected. In the pursuit of being affirmed and loved, we often get side-tracked into believing false narratives such as:

- Life is all about me.
- This drug or this drink will heal my hurts and numb the pain.
- The more partners I have, the more power I hold.
- If only I were skinnier, taller, shorter, smarter, prettier, or more successful.
- I need money, looks, power, prestige, and position to be someone.
- I don't need to answer to anyone.
- I am my own boss.
- I don't have to listen to anyone.
- I can take the easier route to avoid pain.
- I don't need any man to tell me what to do.
- Women are superior to men.
- I need to be strong so no one will ever hurt me again.

I spent too many years believing those lies, and they almost brought about my own death. I kept pursuing them all, but nothing seemed to fill the void inside me. I finally came to the realization that I was better off dead. While I wanted to die on several occasions, I only tried to take my life once. But none of these pursuits and lies can bring about the fulfillment and peace we so desperately desire. Nothing but Christ can fill the void. I know because I tried. I also know because when He came into my life, the void was filled for the first time *and* the last time.

Ultimately, the wounds women carry around will define us, our children, and future generations. We have to make the intentional choice to live a life of purpose, not one based only on what feels good in the moment. *Feelings are not facts.* Allow me to repeat that statement: Feelings are not facts. I struggled with that statement for many years but learned the hard way that it is true. I wanted my feelings to be facts because I needed to be justified. However, my perception was so distorted that I could not make sense of my own feelings. Of course, feelings are essential and God-given, but they are not meant to rule our decision-making. How we feel changes often, so that is not a solid standard to follow. Our twenty-first-century society has adopted a faulty belief system of appealing to our emotions and a demand of "personal rights."

But the good news is that we do not have to be slaves to our wounds. We can stop the infectious disease of resentment, bitterness, unforgiveness, and lack of love from being spread any further to those around us. Life is not about denying our emotions, but acknowledging them and then deciding how to correctly respond—to no longer let circumstances determine how we will respond.

Making a premeditated decision of response is the beneficial choice. We identify the emotion and then direct the appropriate response. We have to base our decisions on truth, not feelings. People's words or actions should not define us, because our wounds no longer define us. In my case, I came to the personal choice that God will define me and that He desires for me to receive His healing for my wounds.

Few people these days want to talk about a relationship with God for fear of being misunderstood or judged, but I cannot leave this opportunity untouched. Too much is at stake in this regard. I was a skeptic when it came to God. I often wondered, *What if this is all just a lie? What if God is not real? If God is really a loving God, why would He allow my innocence to be stolen at five years old? Why or how does God look on while such evil happens? How can a loving God allow this pain to be inflicted upon His creation?*

We hear horrific stories every evening on the news, and we find ourselves asking the age-old, still-unanswered question again and again: Why would a good God allow bad things to happen to good people? In spite of the frequency and number of times the question has been asked, the answer doesn't come because we cannot see into, know, and fully understand the mind and reasoning of a holy, righteous God. The prophet Isaiah spoke to this truth:

> *"For my thoughts are not your thoughts, neither are your ways my ways," declares the Lord. "As the heavens are higher than the earth, so are my ways higher than your ways and my thoughts than your thoughts." (Isaiah 55:8–9 NIV)*

Free will is not selective, but universal and innate. Free will when mishandled breeds bad choices. Bad choices generate bad consequences and repercussions that spill over into the lives of others, causing a ripple effect in the present and also into future generations.

For me, I struggled for so long to wrap my mind around a loving God who would allow for such suffering, but what I finally concluded is this: The *power* of God's healing and redemption in my own life has caused me to embrace the *sovereignty* of God, to accept that He alone knows best beyond what I can see.

> *To have faith is to be sure of the things we hope for, to be certain of the things we cannot see. (Hebrews 11:1 GNT)*

HOPE AND HEALING FOR THE BROKENHEARTED

I want to offer you some simple steps of what I did to surrender to Christ, give up my past, receive help, healing, and hope, to walk into the future God had for me all along.

1. Admit that you are wounded and must have God's help to heal those wounds.

If we claim we have no sin, we are only fooling ourselves and not living in the truth. But if we confess our sins to him, he is faithful and just to forgive us our sins and to cleanse us from all wickedness. (1 John 1:8–9)

Confess your sins to each other and pray for each other so that you may be healed. (James 5:16)

2. Decide to let go of fear, despair, bitterness, anger, and hatred.

Get rid of all bitterness, rage, anger, harsh words, and slander, as well as all types of evil behavior. Instead, be kind to each other, tenderhearted, forgiving one another, just as God through Christ has forgiven you. (Ephesians 4:31–32)

3. Go back through your past history to reveal the original source of the harmful, negative emotions.

Take an inventory of your past and determine how the wound began. Who was the offender? What did he/she/they do? How did it affect you? Examples would be divorce, alcoholism, a controlling relationship, an obsessive-compulsive parent, death, or abuse.

If I was ever going to get out of the cycle of blaming others, I had to face myself and confess my part in everything. I had to accept that I could not change anyone else but me. I only had the power to invite change into *my* own life.

When our initial wounds occur, we develop negative coping skills. Without anything or anyone to change that mindset, we often carry those throughout life and, as the wounds fester and become infected, we start to infect everyone else along the way. As difficult as accepting and owning up to your part of any of your past may be, this has to be done. This step is crucial in moving on.

One way to communicate this concept is in one situation where you were wounded, your part was only ten percent, but in another, yours was ninety percent of the issue. Getting real about your involvement in your own hurts does not mean taking all of the blame or none, but rather facing the facts of what you may have done and owning up to your part.

This concept is often seen in a nasty divorce. Both husband and wife lay one-hundred percent of the blame at the feet of the other. Then as soon as another relationship is started, that spouse's twenty, fifty, or eighty percent is put back in play in the new relationship, and the new infection from the old wound begins to be targeted toward a different person.

This is exactly why you find men who, after many failed relationships, will say, "All women are crazy," or a woman who comes to the conclusion, like I did, of "All men are idiots." Once we can get honest and admit, "This is the toxicity I tend to bring to the table in relationships" and start to address that for ourselves, life can begin to change.

4. Treat the wound.

If we keep playing the blame game or seeking retaliation, we can never get well. We have to extend forgiveness. We often come to believe that what has happened to us is unforgiveable. Yet unforgiveness gives us a false sense of power, which translates to anger, bitterness, or even hatred. Forgiveness releases us from the bondage of the past to free us from the infection of bitterness, anger, revenge, and the victim role. Forgiveness and God's love can heal the infection.

> *He heals the brokenhearted and bandages their wounds. (Psalm 147:3)*

Choosing to not forgive people is like taking them hostage. As the bitterness sets in, we abduct the person and tie them to the chair of our offense. The hideout where we keep our hostages is our own heart, covertly tucked away. Most people will never know that we are keeping others locked up in there.

But here is the horrible plot twist: The person or people we won't forgive are not actually who is tied up in the chair after all. They are not actually the hostages. We are the hostages. We are the ones bound up. We are the ones in hiding. Our offender is out walking the streets in total freedom—rarely, if ever, thinking about us. But he/she is on our mind daily.

So, the *only* cure for unforgiveness is forgiveness.

The power of forgiveness came for me when I was able to write my dad a letter telling him I was sorry for all the things I had done wrong, such as disobeying his authority, taking my mom and him for granted, and other hurtful behaviors. As much as I could have blamed him for many things, God impressed upon *my* heart to look at only my part. I closed my letter by asking Bill to forgive me, thanking him for teaching me a good work ethic, and telling him I loved him.

After I wrote the letter and sent it, I felt so free. Because I had released him and me from the past. I owned up to my part and gave God the rest. Bill never called or spoke with me about the letter, but I did ask him if he received it and he said he had. Does his lack of acknowledgment and response sadden me because the relationship could not be fully restored? Of course. But I took the action God required of me for freedom. I did my part. I am no longer responsible for the results. God is now in control.

Again, here are Jesus' words on this issue:

> *"So if you are presenting a sacrifice at the altar in the Temple and you suddenly remember that someone has something against you, leave your sacrifice there at the altar. Go and be reconciled to that person. Then come and offer your sacrifice to God." (Matthew 5:23–24)*

Look at what Paul said about relationships and note his qualifiers to allow for taking care of only your part:

> *If it is possible, as far as it depends on you, live at peace with everyone. (Romans 12:18 NIV)*

A crucial part of healing is acceptance of our wounds. No more denial, blame, or hiding. We may never know this side of Heaven why certain things have happened to us. My heart is broken all over again every time I think about how my innocence was stolen at such a young age. No child should ever have to go through that. But so many things in this life are consequences of living in a fallen and broken world of sin.

Let's close this section with more of Jesus' teaching that is paradoxical to the ways of this world.

> *"You have heard the law that says the punishment must match the injury: 'An eye for an eye, and a tooth for a tooth.' But I say, do not resist an evil person! If someone slaps you on the right cheek, offer the other cheek also. If you are sued in court and your shirt is taken from you, give your coat, too. If a soldier demands that you carry his gear for a mile, carry it two miles. Give to those who ask, and don't turn away from those who want to borrow.*
>
> *"You have heard the law that says, 'Love your neighbor' and hate your enemy. But I say, love your enemies! Pray for those who persecute you! In that way, you will be acting as true children of your Father in heaven. For he gives his sunlight to both the evil and the good, and he sends rain*

on the just and the unjust alike. If you love only those who love you, what reward is there for that? Even corrupt tax collectors do that much. If you are kind only to your friends, how are you different from anyone else? Even pagans do that." (Matthew 5:38–47)

In a word,

what I'm saying is,

Grow up.

You're kingdom subjects.

Now live like it.

Live out your God-created identity.

Live generously and

graciously toward others,

the way God lives toward you.

Matthew 5:48 MSG

CHAPTER EIGHT

Define Yourself by the Power of Christ, Not the Wounds of Your Past

First, let's define the word *victim*. A victim is someone who is:

- Adversely affected physically, mentally, emotionally, or spiritually by a force or agent
- Subjected to oppression, hardship, or mistreatment
- Tricked or duped by an individual or a group

Some behaviors or symptoms demonstrated by victims are:

- Trauma
- PTSD
- Self-harm
- Suicidal ideation
- Lack of trust
- Difficulty forgiving
- Depression
- Anxiety
- Lack of coping skills
- Memory lapses and/or gaps
- Unsubstantiated fear of impending danger, evil, pain
- Expressions of despair, dismay, panic, suspicion, timidity, or uneasiness

THE DANGERS OF VICTIMIZATION

With that information in mind, I want to present a Christian worldview, with my first statement being that an environment that embraces victimization can never live in harmony with the power of the Gospel of Christ. When we create and foster a victim mentality, we discount the truth of God's Word that transforms and changes lives. Far too many in our society today want to exploit victims and encourage avoidance of the core issues, instead of equipping them with the victory over their adversity. Sadly, this is also seen even in the Western church. Spiritual leaders should take caution in cultivating *any* environment that fosters cultural victimization over spiritual victory.

To be clear, we must of course recognize and deal with the reality of what anyone has suffered and allow time for healing. My point is not to create a lifestyle and adopt a mindset of being a victim. If you were abused, molested, raped, bullied, or harmed in another way, I am so sorry. I understand. I empathize. I know your pain. That pain is real, and I do not desire to diminish your experience in any way. What I do want to express are the dangers of allowing those emotions to go unchecked and not dealt with. They will wreak havoc on your life as they did on mine.

> *Dear brothers and sisters, if another believer is overcome by some sin, you who are godly should gently and humbly help that person back onto the right path. And be careful not to fall into the same temptation yourself. Share each*

other's burdens, and in this way obey the law of Christ. If you think you are too important to help someone, you are only fooling yourself. You are not that important. (Galatians 6:1–3)

The L*ORD* *is close to the brokenhearted; he rescues those whose spirits are crushed. (Psalm 34:18)*

We disempower victims when all we can talk about is how bad their life is and never address how to seek freedom. This mindset is happening in so many areas of our culture. But we must ask the question: While most victims *feel* powerless, why would anyone want victims to *stay* powerless?

The sad and simple answer is because they can be easy prey who are easily influenced. They can be manipulated for others' purposes and to further others' agendas. Because they have an ax to grind on an issue or a vendetta against someone (or sometimes an entire segment of the population), they are offered a false sense of power by handing over a megaphone that actually allows that power to fall into the wrong hands and be used for someone else's platform, often totally unrelated to the victim's original issue. For an easy example, how many times have we seen a very real victim who has suffered be used as a front on a crowdfunding site for another's greed?

Women who are wounded at the hands of men often develop a "hear me roar" mentality and look to destroy *anyone* in their path. Today we see this dynamic expressed by extreme feminists. When we play into the victim mindset, we use the circumstance to foster an excuse to *not* change. Blaming others, rightfully earned or not, never becomes about taking ownership to heal a wound. We end up giving all the power right back to the one who inflicted the wound, because bitterness, anger, depression, and other negative behaviors rule the heart.

Victimization often fosters an environment that plays into certain ideologies and religious nuances, and feigns kindness and empathy. If we really want to help a victim, we will want to empower them to overcome their past to live *better* lives than ever before, not keep them living out of a wounded spirit.

When we fall victim to someone else's sin, we often give the perpetrator more power by *staying* the victim to *their* original wound. What we should be talking about is the empowerment that occurs when victims demonstrate bravery and courage by facing head-on the tough issue of deciding to seek healing. To talk about what is required of someone to overcome an inflicted wound. Part of becoming emotionally mature is working through these issues that have defined us for many years.

To say, "Hi, I'm Tonya, a recovering alcoholic" is simply not enough. Better to say, "Hi, I'm Tonya, and I demonstrated courage to determine what kept me in bondage to alcohol and to break the family cycle of alcoholism." To say, "Hi, I'm Tonya, a survivor of childhood sexual assault" is not enough. Better to say, "Hi, I'm Tonya, and I demonstrated courage and bravery to work through the trauma of childhood sexual assault that took me down a path of self-hatred, bitterness, and anger, and fostered an environment that told me to stay a victim to all men."

Continuing to operate out of a wounded spirit can cause us to doubt God and His goodness. And that is exactly what the enemy of God (Satan) wants us to do. When we don't believe God is good, we stay victims and see no hope, living in a cycle of defeat.

While we can remain a victim forever, we need to instead become survivors. A survivor is someone who continues to function or prosper in *spite* of opposition, hardship, or setbacks. The next step is to be an overcomer, someone who conquers and defeats an obstacle or issue—who succeeds in dealing with or gaining self-control over some problem or difficulty.

The opposite of a victim is a survivor. A survivor can then become an overcomer.

Here are some questions to answer in dealing with your wound: (Be as honest and specific as possible.)

1. Who wounded me?
2. What wound or wounds were created in me?
3. How did the offense affect me?
4. What part, if any, did I play in the offense?
5. Who do I need to forgive?
6. What steps can I take to experience freedom?

Eleanor Roosevelt once said, "You gain strength, courage and confidence by every experience in which you really stop to look fear in the face. You are able to say to yourself, 'I have lived through this horror. I can take the next thing that comes along.' You must do the thing you think you cannot do."[1] Courage can be defined as the quality of mind or spirit that enables a person to face difficulty, danger, or pain, without fear. Courage is having valor and guts, producing heroism, fortitude, endurance, and backbone.

> *Be strong and let your heart take courage, All you who wait for the LORD. (Psalm 31:24 NASB)*

Because I have personally experienced the life changing power of the cross, I want to be a courageous overcomer that inspires others to live a life of freedom. Succumbing to all the whys of my adversity would have been so easy to do, to just give up, but I wanted to ensure that courage and intentionality were part of my testimony of God's redemption in my life. We must stand out and be the city on the hill. We are called to let our lights shine and that requires courage.

> *"You are the light of the world—like a city on a hilltop that cannot be hidden. No one lights a lamp and then puts it under a basket. Instead, a lamp is placed on a stand, where it gives light to everyone in the house. In the same way, let your good deeds shine out for all to see, so that everyone will praise your heavenly Father." (Matthew 5:14– 16)*

COMMITTING TO COURAGE

There is a very real war on women today, most particularly in the biblical dynamic and definition of femininity. We live in a very confused world where media outlets and talk show hosts will speak out on behalf of the horrors of the #metoo movement, but then remain silent as innocent children are being objectified on readily available porn sites as victims of human sex trafficking. There is most certainly a double standard.

On the subject of abortion, as another example, the focus is on rights and politics, while women who have undergone this horror silently grieve, needing love and redemption. We can't allow culture, religion, politics, or tradition to be used to perpetuate violence and oppression of the weak and the unborn. We should most certainly question and place a spotlight on practices that are unjust or harmful. We need to save other women's lives and to speak out about the suffering of women and their children. If we are to leave behind a legacy of purpose, we will have to display courage.

Courage is the opposite of fear. I know this because my entire life was fear-based for too many years. We can actually learn to live our lives in fear, with constantly high-strung emotions, rapid heart rates, shallow breathing, and even bouts of paralysis. Experiencing fear can greatly impact our view of life and our confidence levels, and can sabotage our potential for personal growth.

Fear is one of the primary weapons that Satan uses to isolate and neutralize us. While fear weakens, courage strengthens. Mark Twain said, "Courage is resistance to fear, mastery of fear, not absence of fear."[2] Inaction breeds doubt and fear, while action breeds confidence and courage. Dale Carnegie stated, "If you want to conquer fear, don't sit at home and think about it. Go out and get busy."[3]

> *Wait for the LORD; Be strong and let your heart take courage; Yes, wait for the Lord. (Psalm 27:14 NASB)*

To "take heart" means to be confident or courageous in a difficult situation.

> *When I am afraid, I put my trust in you. In God, whose word I praise—in God I trust and am not afraid. What can mere mortals do to me? (Psalm 56:3–4 NIV)*

We need to live courageously because that is the spirit God has given us.

> *For God has not given us a spirit of fear and timidity, but of power, love, and self-discipline. (2 Timothy 1:7)*

We can choose to live a life of purpose by knowing that life is short and we aren't guaranteed tomorrow so we must make the most of today. We are called to rise up and combat the damaging narrative from the world through courage, intentionality, and living out our purpose through God's calling. We can make a difference across our nation and around the world by being the voice for people that speaks for hope, intentionality, and meaningful legacies.

> *"And who knows whether you have not come to the kingdom for such a time as this?" (Esther 4:14 ESV)*

Our future generations are counting on us to be the next greatest generation. Ronald Reagan stated in one of his most iconic speeches, "Freedom is never more than one generation away from extinction. We didn't pass it to our children in the bloodstream. It must be fought for, protected, and handed on for them to do the same, or one day we will spend our sunset years telling our children and our children's children what it was once like in the United States where men were free."[4]

The enemy of God hates us and has his sights set on our kids and grandkids. He will do anything possible to take them out through media, technology, social media, the celebrity culture, and parental complacency. In the name of "freedom of speech" and the new definition of "tolerance," which has ironically become intolerance, we have abdicated our responsibility to both the next generation as well as our nation's heritage.

One of the by-products of expressing and displaying courage in our life is developing resilience. To be courageous and resilient, we must also develop healthy coping skills to properly deal with adversity. One of the commonalities we find in kids or women who end up in correctional facilities is that their hurts and frustrations with life have resulted in their having no coping skills. Therefore, a total lack of resistance to external pressure or harmful influence. Part of the reasoning behind the lack of resilience is that they were never taught coping skills, which in turn reduces their ability to be resilient.

My husband, Rich, is resilient even though he was deemed the "black sheep" of his family, has dealt with divorce, and has experienced failure after failure. He never stops loving. He never gives up. He has told me that he would never allow anyone to fail, if it was up to him, including his own enemies. Rich believes everyone deserves a chance to succeed. Why? Because he did and he understands the power of resilience.

An intentional life has purpose, discipline, and vision. We often have good intentions, but for varied reasons we don't follow through. In James 5:12, we are told, "Let your yes be yes and your no be no." To live an intentional life, we must:

- Be a person of our word
- Always follow through
- Right the wrongs when it is in our power to act
- Be humble

If we don't have a plan, life can easily get away from us and we can be knocked off course. God has always operated in an intentional manner. In Job 42:2, Job says of God after his suffering, "I know you can do all things, and that no purpose of yours can be thwarted" (NIV).

> *"I make known the end from the beginning, from ancient times, what is still to come. I say, 'My purpose will stand, and I will do all that I please.'"* (Isaiah 46:10 NIV)

Here are some action steps for intentionality:

- Make a plan
- Work the plan
- Monitor the plan
- Adjust the plan
- Persevere in the plan

Today, as in the days of Jesus, we are in a spiritual battle, and we must recognize our need and call to armor up. We must recognize the Enemy's tactics and gear up.

> *And that about wraps it up. God is strong, and he wants you strong. So take everything the Master has set out for you, well-made weapons of the best materials. And put them to use so you will be able to stand up to everything the Devil throws your way. This is no afternoon athletic contest that we'll walk away from and forget about in a couple of hours. This is for keeps, a life-or-death fight to the finish against*

> *the Devil and all his angels. Be prepared. You're up against far more than you can handle on your own. Take all the help you can get, every weapon God has issued, so that when it's all over but the shouting you'll still be on your feet. Truth, righteousness, peace, faith, and salvation are more than words. Learn how to apply them. You'll need them throughout your life. God's Word is an indispensable weapon. In the same way, prayer is essential in this ongoing warfare. Pray hard and long. Pray for your brothers and sisters. Keep your eyes open. Keep each other's spirits up so that no one falls behind or drops out. (Ephesians 6:10–18 MSG)*

THE VULNERABILITY OF TRUST

All good fairy tales and film classics have happy endings, so this book must have the iconic knight-in-shining-armor rescuing the damsel-in-distress, right? I have shared my story, and you now know how difficult it was for me to trust a man and make the decision to take down my emotional walls. This particular decision was life-changing in my marriage.

For years, I have worked with women in our community and our church to teach them life skills. One particular girl I mentored got involved in some, let's say, illegal activity, and I was asked to testify about her boyfriend at a trial. I agreed to help the DA's office, and I was briefly prepped to be put on the witness stand.

When I was sworn in, I was extremely nervous. The prosecuting attorney asked me how I knew the defendant. I responded by saying the young lady whom I had mentored came to me concerned about the defendant's involvement in a string of robberies. Apparently, I was not supposed to say "string of robberies." I was to only use the singular form, "robbery." The judicial court system does not like to be biased about a criminal's past, so each crime is tried separately. Immediately, the defense attorney asked to approach the bench. After a brief exchange, they excused and escorted me into a private room. I didn't know what was happening and was now somewhat scared.

As I waited for the attorney's assistant to speak, the prosecuting attorney—the one I was trying to help—walked into the other room, not knowing I was in the adjacent room, and told the people waiting there that I had blown the whole case for them. Immediately, I could feel my blood boiling, and I got up and walked into their room. You should have seen the look on his face when he saw me and realized I had overheard what he just said.

Angry, I stated, "That is not fair for you to say! I was just doing what I was told and trying to help you!" I then burst into tears and went back into the little room where I had been waiting. The assistant came in, apologized, and told me the judge had declared a mistrial. I, of course, had a million questions, and she basically said we were going back to square one. They told me they would get in touch with me for the next trial.

When I got to my car, I was crying hysterically and called Rich to tell him what happened. He asked for the attorney's name and phone number. I asked why, and he replied, "Because I'm going to call him." I responded, "I don't think so, Rich. Let's just let it go." But Rich was adamant about calling, so I gave him the number. He called, and then called me back. "I took care of it," he said simply. He then told me to get in touch with them and set up a time for me to go to their office so they could apologize to me—in person.

I really did not want to go through that. I was planning a big fortieth surprise birthday party for Rich, and his family was coming to town in two days. I didn't have time for this drama. I told Rich I just wanted to be done and move on, to which he asked, "Tonya, do you know what kind of guts it took to call the county attorney and tell him he would apologize to my wife?" He continued, "I told him he did not properly do his job, and if it was anyone's fault, it was theirs for not prepping you correctly. He is probably running a background check on me as we speak."

I laughed hard. And then I started crying again. About a half hour later, I received a call from the assistant to arrange a meeting in the DA's office the following morning. I reluctantly said I would come. That night, I couldn't sleep because I knew my mistake would likely be all over the local paper in the morning. Sure enough, and true to their reputation, I was front page news. The paper over-simplified and misclassified me as the girl's "friend." *Great, now I'm going to have every drug lord in the city after me!* I thought.

Furious, I went to my meeting and was greeted by the chief attorney, the prosecuting attorney, and his assistant. They told me they had tried to get a retraction from our local paper, but to no avail. They then apologized for what took place the day before and were gracious and humble about it. While it was a kind gesture, the fear of the drug lords was still very real to me. The good news is that no one ever stalked me or my family and we were never threatened.

I love this story because nobody had ever stood up for me the way Rich did in that situation. When I was five and sexually abused, having that kind of protection would have changed the course of my life for the good. Unfortunately, that did not happen. Throughout my younger years, I lacked protection. But after twenty years of hiding my near-fatal wound, I finally had the knight I had so longed for and wanted.

To be clear, Rich was there the whole time, but I often rejected his efforts to protect me. I believed I was the one in control. I thought I was the only one who could protect me and was blinded by my own iniquities. I couldn't yet see that I already had the knight I had wanted all along. But here's the game changer—I had to be *willing* to be rescued. Not weak-willed and incapable, but rather vulnerable. Being vulnerable is the willingness to admit to being wounded and in need of help.

As I previously stated, that takes courage, something we desperately lack in our world today. Most want to take the easy way out and hide or indulge in temporary fixes. As women, if we take the time and find the courage to receive God's healing and build our husbands up the way God intended, we can have the fairy-tale marriage.

I realize you might have been hurt at the hands of a man more times than you can count. Maybe it's the guy you are with right now. He abuses you in one way or another. Please know you have a choice in how you will proceed in the relationship. You can choose to get help for yourself and work on the healing of your own individual wounds, or you can stay in that insane cycle of chaos. True wisdom comes from putting knowledge into action. You can know everything you need to do to change your situation and be educated with a gazillion degrees, but until you put the knowledge you have into *action*, real help and hope will not be found.

Are you willing to take the first step in your family and sphere of influence to fill your mind and home with positive messages about masculinity and femininity? We have a voice. We can use our knowledge and wisdom to leave a legacy for our children and grandchildren that will impact the rest of our lives and theirs.

Countless articles and books have been written on the lack of leadership from men in our society. We know we are in a cultural crisis with the absence of a male figure in over half of our homes, some where he is literally not there and others where he is there but not truly present. Because of this, there is an urgency to help our communities become places where real men have a position of leadership and importance. Women have created an environment of superiority, causing the emasculation of men. So as women we have a great opportunity to make our society and the world a better place by how we empower others, *all* others, because we have been healed.

When we live life operating out of a wounded spirit, we will eventually wound others. As the old saying goes, "Hurt people hurt people." We have to learn to work together and build each other up. Of course, this does not mean you will be exempt from being backstabbed or hurt by others, but are you going to let others' actions define you? Or are you going to get back up, dust yourself off, and use courage to persevere?

Empowering others begins in our homes, but then reaches out from there into our community. This is how legacies begin—by someone choosing to get outside of themselves and live a life of courage, intentionality, and love.

"This is my command—

be strong and courageous!

Do not be afraid or discouraged.

For the Lord your God

is with you wherever you go."

Joshua 1:9

CHAPTER NINE

Devote Your Life to Inspiring Others by Expressing Courage

None of us know our final hour here on earth. We see this fact time and again in the lives of our families and friends who have suddenly lost loved ones. My mom's death was sudden. Dave's death was a shock too. Often we do not see death coming, and there will be times when we are blindsided. After I lost my mom, I had so many regrets. I wished I could have told her how sorry I was for how I had treated her on so many occasions. I have spent many days in the pit of guilt over all the things I did *not* get to say or do. This thought grieves my soul. But it's done. And even today, the feeling of regret hasn't gone away. There are still many days I wish I could talk with my mom.

On August 23, 1997, I didn't just lose my mom. I also lost my dad. My mother's death pushed him farther away from our family, and he never recovered. Even up until his own death, he never really wanted to be around us. I lost my mother and the only man I ever knew as a father. I do not understand why, but I have to believe God has a purpose for it all.

Here's the question I have for you: "Are you ready?" If you or someone you love died today, would you have any regrets? About anything done or said? About anything *not* done or said? How would you live life differently if you knew you had just a short time to live? When someone is dying, you never hear them talk about accumulating more wealth or power. What almost every single one of them wants to talk about are the relationships with their loved ones.

LEAVING A LASTING LEGACY

The presence of a deadline to life often creates a time for reconciliation and words that some have waited years to hear. For those of us who know Jesus, we will be reunited again in Heaven, but ultimately we have to take a moment to reflect on how we are living life *right now.*

When the day of your funeral arrives, what else is there to evaluate other than the legacy left behind to your family and the generations to come?

Most people think death will not happen to them anytime soon, so they put off the important things of life. There is a reason the fear of death is one of the top fears. So people avoid thinking about it or dealing with it. Having no control over death frightens them. That fear has led to a false mindset that, if you do not think about death, it won't happen to you. However, we know the truth: death comes to us all.

The church or funeral home is filled with people who gather to pay their respects to the life the person lived. Some will get up and speak about the impact made on them. But imagine for a moment that a large U-Haul trailer is hitched to the back of your hearse. The person officiating your funeral announces to everyone that you have left behind some parting gifts. Some of these gifts are so priceless that no one can put a value on them—gifts of faith, hope, and love. But others are gifts of anger, bitterness, and silence. Have you ever lost a family member or friend, and it was hard for you to come up with positive aspects of their life because so much was covered in darkness? Personally, I do not want to come to the end of my life only to reflect back on any harmful gifts left to *anyone*.

If you know you have just been surviving your entire life—if you have lived a life defined by your wounds—don't you want more for yourself and your family between now and the end of life?

What kind of legacy will you leave behind when you're gone?

What will people say about how you lived?

What will you have left behind in their hearts and minds?

What will your children and spouse say about how you impacted their lives?

What will your coworkers say about how you impacted them?

Is your life filled with purpose?

If not, what steps can you take *right now* to change?

I encourage you to think about these things, about these questions I have asked, that I have had to face and answer for myself. That's why I know how to ask these of you. Facing these questions is difficult, but it forces us to reflect on what we are actually doing with our lives and the time we have left.

A life of self-indulgence is quickly forgotten, but a life of purpose and intentionality is one passed down and remembered for generations to come. There have been too many days, months, and years in my own journey when I asked, *Why me? Why was I sexually abused at five? Why couldn't my innocence have been protected? Why wasn't I good enough for the men in my life? Why did my mom have to die? Why did I have to lose two babies? Why would a loving God allow so much suffering in my life?*

Finally, it all came down to whether I was going to be a victim of the why-mes and all my affliction, or whether I was going to trust God. As I approached this challenge of faith on my journey, I came to a crossroads and made a conscious decision to trust Him.

> *And we know that for those who love God all things work together for good, for those who are called according to his purpose. (Romans 8:28 ESV)*

Often, on the other side of this coin, I have questioned how God could ever use someone like me to make a difference in the world when I have had such a pitiful past. But God says He will use *all* things for good. The problem was that the victim in me was interfering with God's trying to bring the good out of my pain. I finally gave up and gave in, trusting Him and having faith to believe that He will use my pain and suffering for others in His greater purpose. I have a testimony of hope today only because I put my trust and faith in Jesus Christ.

Because of this decision, my testimony is really not my story at all, but God's story of hope in my life, a journey of healing and trusting who He says He is and choosing to live my life based on His Word, His ways, and His will. I was constantly disappointed when I had control of my life or gave that to someone else. I have yet to be disappointed in my decision to give my life to Christ.

Being a woman who has struggled with sexual abuse, alcohol abuse, promiscuous behavior, and a distorted belief system has given me insight and understanding to many behaviors that others often see as completely irrational and just plain stupid. Often, "normal people" cannot understand the thinking involved in these actions. But God has given me opportunities to work with women, through our church and community, who are often in these crisis situations. I have had the blessing of mentoring many through difficult seasons of life. I get to use my past, coupled with my faith and maturity in Christ, to give them coping skills that can lead them out of bondage. Like a beggar who found a banquet, I can now lead others to the table.

Rich and I know firsthand the effects of addiction. We are both recovering addicts. Today, more and more people are living with addiction because of their lack of coping skills. Our experience causes us to have empathy for families that are in crisis with addiction. We can then help them in their journey toward recovery. Almost every family will deal with addiction in one way or another, and God has allowed Rich and me to be vessels of hope as others learn how to walk through that specific adversity.

Beyond our empathy for addiction support, we also can empathize with those who care for children with special needs. Three of our five children were born with health challenges. Our oldest daughter is hearing impaired. Our oldest son has a speech impediment. Our youngest daughter had a seizure disorder. We have experienced many seasons of life dealing with the medical unknown. For example, we didn't know why our oldest daughter had hearing loss, and we were unsure if she might become completely deaf. We spent many nights praying that God would allow her to keep her hearing in her other ear, and many nights in tears praying she would not have to endure any more teasing from children.

On many occasions, our son experienced relentless teasing because of his speech problem. Bullying is devastating, for the child and the parent. He spent seven years in speech therapy, had several thousand dollars of appliances put into his mouth, and still has seasons where his speech is challenged. However, God has blessed our son with such grace and mercy for people who are considered misfits and castoffs.

Our youngest daughter had a seizure disorder. Nine years of ups and downs, trying to control these episodes, classified as idiopathic, was like riding an emotional roller coaster every day of our lives. That time was frustrating and frightening. Several times, I wondered if she would ever live a normal life. I was so scared of the damage the seizures were doing, and I did not know what the long-term effects would be. When they came on her, we never knew how long each seizure would last, if we would end up at the hospital again, or if she might die. And we had no choice except to endure them.

God has allowed Rich and me to use our adversity to help others who have kids with special needs. Sometimes people just need to know they are not alone in their crisis. So many people experience isolation through trials, and we know our experiences are to encourage people to know that others have also walked these difficult roads and survived. God answered our prayers, and our oldest has not lost any more hearing and our youngest daughter has been declared seizure-free.

Sadly, we have experienced much death in our family. We had one miscarriage at eight weeks and another at sixteen weeks. Losing a loved one quickly provides the perspective that life is fragile. What's more, death causes you to be mindful of the lasting impact we can have on the lives of others. My mother's death caused me to see how I had to make the most of every day because I did not know when my last one would be.

Yet, I use those regrets to spur me on to always say what needs to be said, so when I do face another death, I will know I have done all I could to have a right relationship with everyone in my life. Rich and I have been able to walk beside friends who have lost babies, parents, siblings, and children. While we do not always know what to say, the ministry of presence is sometimes more powerful than words in a time of great need.

While we would never choose any of these crises we have had to deal with, they have all allowed Rich and me to grow stronger and closer as a couple. Of course, like most all marriages, we have experienced the fights and sleepless nights with one of us on the couch. We have had heated discussions on parenting, holidays, family traditions, and even manners. We have dealt with the intense pressures of financial hardships. We have had discussions about physical intimacy and the periodic lack of romance. We have had honest talks about our disappointments in each other. And yes, there have even been a few extreme situations when we used the "D" word (divorce). I never recommend that, but for the sake of being real with you, as I have been committed to from page one, you must know we have faced several tough seasons and come through on the other side.

Today, Rich and I often joke about the fact that we really didn't start liking each other until about ten years into our marriage. Although being husband and wife will never be easy, we have learned to rely on prayer and our faith in God to walk us through the challenges of life. And I am glad to tell you that we could not be more happily married today.

If you look at any statistics, our marriage was destined to fail. All the odds were stacked against us, but God granted us healing for our individual wounds. Through that, we could then bring our individuality to the marriage and create oneness, fulfilling God's original design for marriage. As cliché as this might sound, Rich completes me. He is the most amazing husband and father. He protects us, loves us, and invests in us. I am so blessed. Rich is my best friend. He's my calm in the storm.

Today when I think of Rich, I get emotional because I reflect on what would have happened if I had given up and refused to change and receive God's healing. Gratefully, we can see the miracles that God has done in our marriage. Our marriage today is better than any fairy tale. Not because of anything we achieved, but only because of the grace of God. We allowed Him to work in our lives and heal our wounds so we could be effective for Christ and His purpose.

Rich and I are a team. When we surrendered our lives to Christ and chose to follow Him wholeheartedly, we did not give up anything; we gained everything.

BEAUTY FROM ASHES

God has taken my and Rich's pain and suffering to bring forth beauty from ashes. Only God can take something so broken and damaged and bring healing for His glory.

We all have a purpose, so embracing what we are called to do is vital to healing. However, I have often found myself asking, *Do I have what it takes? Am I good enough? How can God use someone like me with such a pitiful past to make a difference in the world?* When we are in victim mode, we never recognize that our pain has purpose. I often told the Lord I didn't want my pain and suffering to be for nothing. Thinking I could possibly make sense of it all to one day help others helped me. However, the Enemy wants you to believe God is a punishing Father who whispers, "This is just your lot in life, so suck it up and be miserable."

I decided that for the rest of my life, I would use my story to inspire others to a life a freedom and hope. If you think about anyone who inspires you, it will never be someone walking around emotionally wounded in despair. That inspiration will be someone who has chosen to overcome and is living courageously by facing adversity head-on.

Let us be the overcomer who inspires others to live a life of freedom so we leave behind a legacy of courage and intentionality to those who have seen us suffer in our victimization. Take your God-given, Holy Spirit-empowered life and choose courage. We need to witness a generation that is going to rise up and win over the ills and issues of our culture.

Today, children are paying the biggest price for how we live. There are 24.7 million children living without a biological father. One in three do not have access to their father. We are called to protect the most vulnerable and, unfortunately, far too many are being exploited in some way. Children are being sex-trafficked and put on display through horrific acts of pornography. Additionally, we are witnessing a political ideology that embraces the idea of killing a child in the womb right up to birth.

Proverbs 31:8–9 states, "Speak up for those who cannot speak for themselves; ensure justice for those being crushed. Yes, speak up for the poor and helpless, and see that they get justice." This is one of the verses in Scripture that helped me determine my purpose. I wasn't protected at a young age, and I know God has called me to ensure that we work to protect the freedom for our future generations. Who is going to fight for the unborn, sexually abused, orphaned, poor, exploited, and vulnerable? God has most certainly called me to join Him in the battle.

Regardless of where you stand politically, we all know that America is changing rapidly. Daily we have to confront a culture that denies the reality of the Gospel and, indeed, denies the existence of any absolute truth. When we turn a blind eye to the current efforts to repress religious liberty, it is not just an attack on individual freedom, but an assault on the very foundation that has made America the "Land of the Free and Home of the Brave."

If you would have asked me fifteen years ago if I would be doing what I am blessed to be doing today, I would have answered, "There's no way!" But as Mordecai told Queen Esther, "You have been put here for such a time as this." I believe the Lord places us right where we need to be. God always planned for me to be an overcomer through Him. By His grace, the adversity in my life has shaped me into the woman I have become to live out my freedom and influence others to recognize the freedom they have been given as well.

There are times when we have to fight for our freedom, and I believe God has appointed me to this calling for our future generations to preserve the opportunity to freely live out our faith. That is also my career today in the public arena.

Christ has delivered me from victim to overcomer to freedom fighter. Only God can take what was meant for evil and use it to influence others for good, as Joseph reminded us in Genesis 50:20.

In 2011, I was introduced to public policy through a group called Concerned Women for America. CWA is the nation's largest women's organization for shaping public policy. This opportunity offered my first view into this arena. And I was quickly astonished at what I found. Many people in our government have used and created laws for their own selfish gain.

I was incensed when I first discovered that lawmakers were abusing their platform in this way when they were elected to protect our freedoms. That realization and revelation began a pilgrimage for me to ensure that my family's legacy did not happen in vain. It inspired me to make certain my grandfather, uncle, husband, and all the other soldiers who sacrificed for our country did not do so in vain. I had been given a call on my life to protect the most vulnerable who were being victimized by dangerous ideologies and to protect our precious freedoms granted to us by those who went before me.

In 2017, I joined Alliance Defending Freedom, the nation's largest Christian legal organization that advocates for the rights of people to freely live out their faith. We focus on what we refer to as "generational wins." This is where I found my heart in being a true justice warrior. I get the honor of standing up in love against injustice. My passion for this movement comes mostly from my upbringing, but also from the Lord, who took my wounds and redeemed them to empower and equip me to help defend His precious children. In my current role as the State Government Relations Director, I have the privilege of helping influence public policy to strengthen families, protect children, and protect believers' rights to freely live out their faith.

Over these past several years, I have come to discover five roadblocks to ensuring we protect our future generations that must be overcome. They are:

1. Fear
2. Complacency
3. Lack of understanding
4. Lack of speaking truth
5. Lack of skills in managing confrontations

In my role, I have seen that many Christ-followers minimize their influence in the culture. We are given the trendy one-liner of "You be you." We live in a post-Christian society where people seek to exchange any of God's truths for lies, never seeing that His truth only protects us. But as a recovering alcoholic with twenty-five years of sobriety, would I still be sober if someone hadn't shared the hope of the Gospel with me? What if they had looked at my life and just said, "Tonya, you be you." That is why Scripture states that God's truth sets us free. The Gospel allows for a loving and grace-filled way to speak truth. The epidemic passivity among people of faith is detrimental to those who are lost, living dangerous lifestyles, and headed toward Hell. Even when biblical truth is present, it is so often watered down to not be "offensive." As the Western church, we have to stop apologizing for our beliefs and embrace the healing power of the cross.

Jesus said plenty on this topic. Here is one example:

> *"Everyone who acknowledges me publicly here on earth, I will also acknowledge before my Father in heaven. But everyone who denies me here on earth, I will also deny before my Father in heaven. Don't imagine that I came to bring peace to the earth! I came not to bring peace, but a sword." (Matthew 10:32–34)*

The public-policy arena involves what has been for, quite a while, considered a dirty word: politicians. Everyone wants to avoid this subject because it is so terribly messy and getting worse. As with all circles in our culture, it is full of sinful people in need of a Savior, just like any workplace environment.

I get excited when I see God's truth prevail. When I get to witness Him transform lives. Shaping public policy has allowed me to use my influence to present His truth on a national scale. I am so passionate about ensuring that protections are in place for future generations. My hope and prayer is that you will *never* underestimate your own ability to influence others. Our *circles* may be different, but our *calling* is the same in Christ. God is responsible for the outcome, but He is asking each of us to be faithful for Him in our generation. There are millions of little "Tonyas" and "insert your own name" out there who need to be protected and hear the hope of the Gospel.

I want to encourage and ask you to stand with me. We cannot allow culture, religion, or tradition to be used to perpetuate violence and oppression of the weak. We must question and call attention to the practices that are unjust and harmful. We need to be about saving others' lives, both physically and spiritually.

We cannot abdicate our responsibility to younger generations and our nation's heritage in the name of "freedom of speech and tolerance." We have to take back the narrative our faith offers and apply the God-given power to protect those who have no voice or cannot protect themselves.

This is our time to make a difference in our nation. Our time to be the voice for families. To speak out for hope, intentionality, and meaningful legacies. We are called to rise up and display courage, intentionality, and our purpose in God's calling.

"What joy for the nation whose God is the Lord,
whose people he has chosen as his inheritance.
The Lord looks down from heaven and sees the
whole human race. From his throne he observes
all who live on the earth. He made their hearts,
so he understands everything they do.
The best-equipped army cannot save a king,
nor is great strength enough to save a warrior.
Don't count on your warhorse
to give you victory—for all its strength,
it cannot save you.
But the Lord watches over those who fear him,
those who rely on his unfailing love."

Psalm 33:12-18

CONCLUSION

Rescued, Redeemed, and Restored

As women, we hold a tremendous amount of power that fundamentally defines family, society, and the nation. We must not underestimate the power we hold. We must also value the way in which we use that power. We must take every opportunity to help breathe life into others. Women are called to be life-givers in so many ways—physically, emotionally, and spiritually. We must be intentional in taking our role to strengthen families, while battling those movements that threaten the family.

We all know our nation is in crisis. Broken families, drug epidemics, crime, lack of education, homelessness, veterans' neglect, and suicide—on and on the list goes. What if we as women put our efforts into working toward answers for these crises instead of marching for "our rights"?

From my personal view, the crisis of feminism today comes from unattended female wounds. Wounds ignored will define you one way or another. And neglected wounds appeal to today's feminist movement ideology and theology. Believing we can control our own lives is a false sense of power and provides a distraction from the real deep-rooted issues.

While the feminist movement was always meant to bring about equality in society in all areas, many wounded women have unfortunately taken it to the extreme and created the battle of the sexes. Women use the voice of power to hide their emotional vulnerability. This reinforces a self-protection mentality which, in turn, causes women to operate out of the wounded spirit trying to prove every man wrong, powerless, and/or ignorant.

Too many women today believe that any sort of submission to any kind of authority is the giving away of power. Women march out of anger, justification, and wounded spirits. And because of our band-wagon culture, some women may not be hurt, but since they have not figured out how to think for themselves, they just go with the crowd. This mindset is equally threatening to godly feminism as too many do not know how to discern truth. This is happening all across college campuses today with the need for "safe zones" and a growing intolerance of common-sense viewpoints.

God's version of feminism is at its core about empowering others to greatness. Jesus said it best: "Love the Lord your God with all your mind, all your heart, and all your soul." All you have to do is take a look at some of the greatest women in history who have championed causes beyond themselves. Why do you suppose the world loved and so mourned Princess Diana? The answer is quite simple: She was a woman who very publicly overcame adversity and used her influence to champion others. Inspiring courage versus fostering victimization in the lives of others is what will change our communities, families, and nation for good.

You want your life to be defined by something more than your wounds. You desire to leave a legacy of great gifts left to others. As women, regardless of our background, issues, and pain, we can give the gift of true feminism and live out a legacy of courage and purpose from this day throughout the rest of our lives.

I pray you will let God work mightily in your life and be rid of the wounds that keep you in chains of guilt and shame. Let God trade His beauty for your ashes, His strength for your fear, His joy for your mourning, and His peace for your despair. If He can do this for me, He can do the same for you.

As I close, I want to invite you to create a personalized version of Isaiah 61:1–3, found on the next page, by writing your name in the blanks provided. God's promises are for anyone who will believe, but then they quickly become personal promises for our lives as we submit and surrender to Him.

"The Spirit of the Sovereign Lord is upon
__________ for the Lord has anointed
__________ to bring good news to the poor.
He has sent __________ to comfort the
brokenhearted and to proclaim that captives
will be released and prisoners will be freed.
He has sent __________ to tell those who
mourn that the time of the Lord's favor has
come, and with it, . . . he will give a crown of
beauty for ashes, a joyous blessing instead
of mourning, festive praise instead of despair.
In __________ righteousness, [he/she] will
be like great oaks that the Lord
has planted for his own glory."

Isaiah 61:1–3 (adapted)

End Notes

[1] "Eleanor Roosevelt Biography," Franklin D. Roosevelt Library and Museum, https://www.fdrlibrary.org/eleanor-roosevelt.

[2] "Mark Twain Quotes," Brainy Quote, https://www.brainyquote.com/quotes/mark_twain_138540.

[3] "Dale Carnegie Quotes," goodreads, https://www.goodreads.com/quotes/402303-if-you-want-to-conquer-fear-don-t-sit-at-home.

[4] "Ronald Reagan Quotes," goodreads, https://www.goodreads.com/quotes/13915-freedom-is-never-more-than-one-generation-away-from-extinction.

About the Author

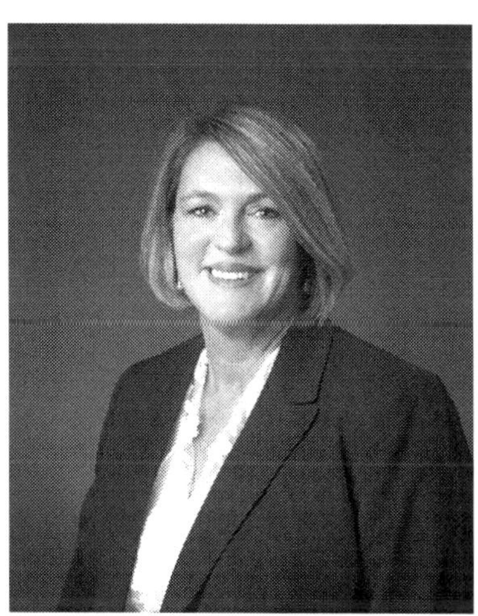

Tonya Shellnutt serves as State Government Relations Director at Alliance Defending Freedom (ADF), the largest religious liberty advocacy organization in the world. ADF exists to keep the legal doors open for the gospel so that we can proclaim the good news and His truth in this culture.

As State Government Relations Director Shellnutt advocates and supports strong pro-family policy upholding the tenants of ADF's strong mission and legal prowess. She regularly convenes policy groups, legislators, and other stakeholders to discuss legislation and strategy to ensure generational wins.

Since joining ADF in 2017, Shellnutt has been working to engage, empower, and protect churches, ministries, and religious institutions across the country. She is committed to safeguarding their religious liberty with legal protections.

Prior to joining ADF, Shellnutt was a small business owner for 15 years and served as State Director for Concerned Women for America (CWA) in both Montana and in South Carolina. While at CWA she focused on faith and family public policy issues. Shellnutt and her husband have been married for 25 years and have five children. Rich and Tonya are extremely passionate about strengthening families and battling the cultural war being waged against traditional families' values. Families are the backbone of our communities, our state, and our country. When we strengthen families, we strengthen communities.

TONYASHELLNUTT.COM

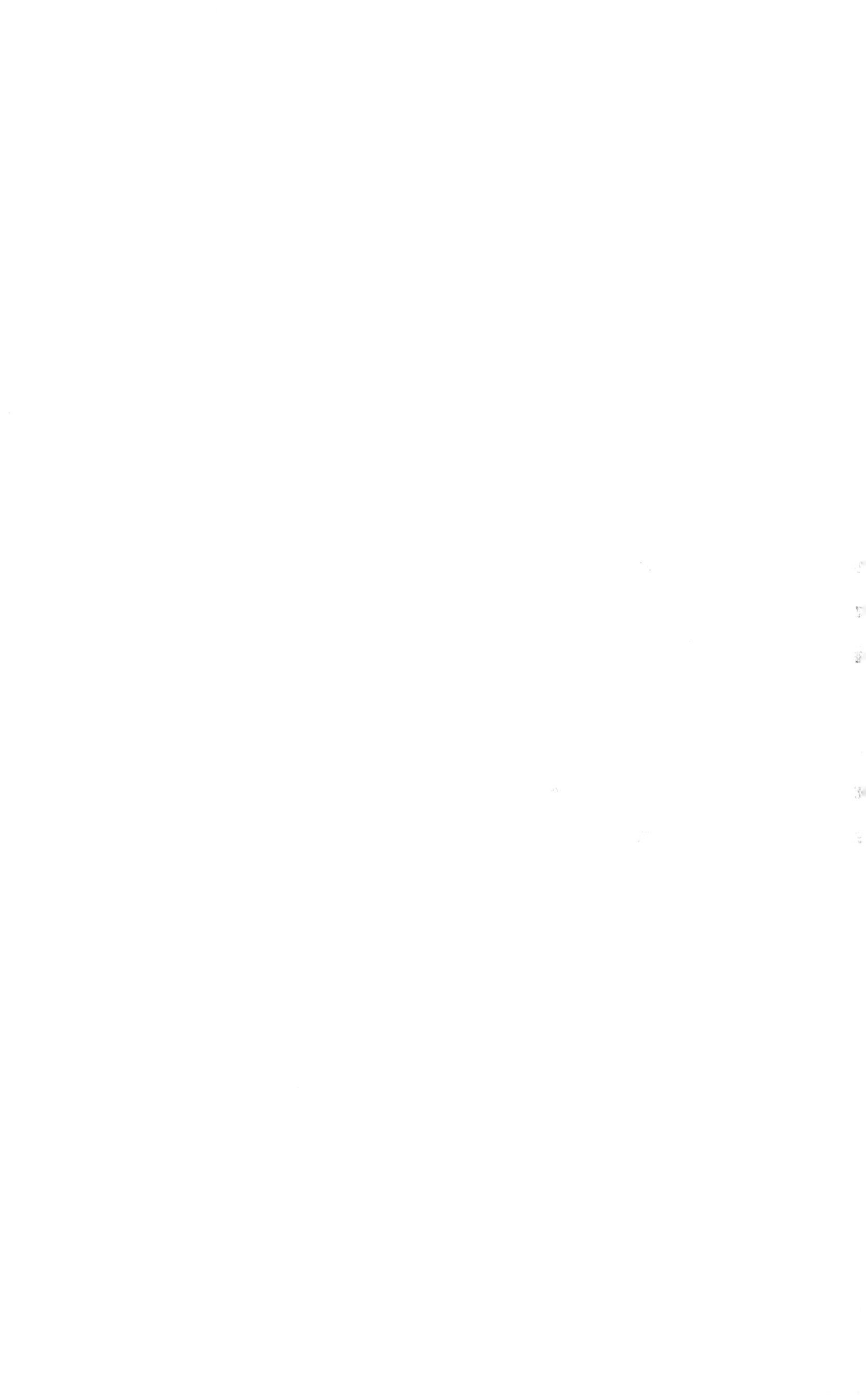

Made in the USA
Columbia, SC
09 February 2024

31096494R00093